Contents

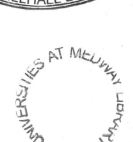

Acknowledgements

CEMACH acknowledges with grateful thanks the contribution made by Dr Mary Macintosh, Medical Director of CEMACH until 30th April 2006, to the Diabetes Programme since its inception in 2001.

Editor

Jo Modder, Clinical Director (Obstetrics)

Authors

- Jo Modder, Clinical Director (Obstetrics)
- Kate Fleming, Senior Data Analyst (until 8th November 2006)
- Dominique Acolet, Clinical Director (Neonatology) – Chapter 12

External commentators

- Kirsty Samuel, Lay Panel Assessor, Yorkshire & Humberside Region
- Sue Roberts, National Clinical Director for Diabetes
- Stephen Walkinshaw, Chair, CEMACH Diabetes Professional Advisory Group
- John Scarpello, Deputy Medical Director, National Patient Safety Agency
- Robert Fraser, Chair, NICE Diabetes in Pregnancy Guideline Development Group
- Patricia Hamilton, President, Royal College of Paediatrics and Child Health

Acknowledgements

Thanks are due to all maternity unit co-ordinators, clinicians and staff who have contributed their time and expertise and without whom this report would not have been possible.

In particular, thanks are due to:

- All Panel Assessors for their extensive and detailed review of medical records during panel enquiries and the significant amount of time contributed to panel meetings.
- All Panel Chairs; for chairing panel enquiries in their region, supporting the CEMACH Regional Managers, and contributing to the recommendations of this report.
- All CEMACH Regional Managers and Assistants for liaising with local clinicians, managing the data collection process, preparing medical records for review and organising panel enquiry meetings.
- Pat Doyle, Head of Department of Epidemiology, London School of Hygiene and Tropical Medicine, for her advice on the statistical analysis of this report.
- Tim Clayton, Medical Statistics Unit, London School of Hygiene and Tropical Medicine, for independent statistical review of this report.
- Gillian Hawthorne, Consultant Diabetes Physician, Newcastle Diabetes Centre, for her contribution to the analysis of enquiry panels' free text comments.
- Oliver Rackham, Consulant Paediatrician, Arrowe Park Hospital, for his contribution to the analysis of cause of death of stillbirths and neonatal deaths.
- Chris Wright, Consultant Paediatric Pathologist, Royal Victoria Infirmary, for his advice regarding the data on post mortem examination.

- Members of the CEMACH Diabetes Professional Advisory Group (chaired by Stephen Walkinshaw) for their support during the Diabetes Programme, and in particular, their advice on the development of data tools and processes of the enquiry, the content of this report and their contribution to the recommendations contained within this report.
- Members of the Neonatal Enquiry Steering Group for their contribution to the development of the Neonatal Enquiry, the content of the neonatal chapter, and their contribution to the neonatal recommendations.
- Peer reviewers of the report (Appendix F).
- Rosie Houston, Assistant Projects Manager, for managing the publication of this report.
- Naufil Alam, Data Analyst; Alison Miller, Programme Director and Midwifery Lead; Shona Golightly, Director of Research and Development; Richard Congdon, CEMACH Chief Executive; and all other staff at CEMACH Central Office for their support and advice during the development of this report.

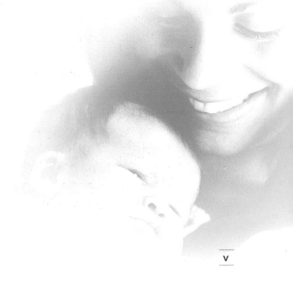

Glossary and abbreviations

AC	Abdominal circumference
ACE inhibitor	Angiotensin-converting enzyme inhibitor; a class of drugs that reduce peripheral arterial resistance by inactivating an enzyme that converts angiotensin I to the vasoconstrictor angiotensin II.
Albuminuria	The presence of albumin in the urine, indicating renal dysfunction
Antenatal	The period of time in pregnancy preceding birth
Antepartum stillbirth	Death of a baby before the onset of labour
Audit	An examination or review that establishes the extent to which a condition, process, or performance conforms to predetermined standards or criteria
Autolysis	Spontaneous disintegration of cells or tissues by autologous enzymes, as occurs after death
Black, Asian and Other minority ethnic group	Term encompassing Black, Asian, Chinese and other ethnic groups as distinct from White ethnic origin
BM	A blood glucose testing strip originally made by the pharmaceutical company Boehringer Mannheim (now Roche). 'BM' is often used to describe any non-laboratory blood glucose test.
BMI	Body Mass Index
Body Mass Index	The body's weight in kilograms divided by the square of the height in metres, used in the assessment of obesity
Caesarean section	Surgical abdominal delivery of the baby
Caesarean section rate	The percentage of births that are by caesarean section
Cardiomegaly	Enlargement of the heart
Cardiotocograph	Graphical representation of electronic monitoring of the fetal heart rate and of uterine contractions. The fetal heart rate is recorded by means of either an external ultrasonic abdominal transducer or a fetal scalp electrode. Uterine contractions are recorded by means of an abdominal pressure transducer.
Case-control study	A study that compares exposure in subjects who have a particular outcome with those who do not
CEMACH	Confidential Enquiry into Maternal and Child Health
Centile	Any of the 99 numbered points that divide an ordered set of scores into 100 parts each of which contains one-hundredth of the total
Childbearing age	Defined as 15 to 44 years
CNST	Clinical Negligence Scheme for Trusts
Confidence interval	A range of values for which there is a 95% chance that it includes the true value.
Confounder	A factor that can bring an alternative explanation to an association observed between an exposure and the outcome of interest
Congenital anomaly	A physical or biochemical malformation which is present at birth
CTG	Cardiotocograph
Early neonatal death	Death of a live born baby occurring less than 7 completed days from the time of birth
Diabetic ketoacidosis	A state of absolute or relative insulin deficiency characterised by hyperglycaemia, dehydration, acidosis and ketosis
Diabetic nephropathy	Kidney dysfunction or disease occurring as a result of diabetes
Diabetic retinopathy	A complication of diabetes affecting the blood vessels in the retina at the back of the eye, which can affect vision. There may be bleeding from retinal vessels (non-proliferative retinopathy) or the development of new abnormal vessels (proliferative retinopathy).
DKA	Diabetic ketoacidosis

Erb's palsy	Injury to the nerve roots of the brachial plexus of an arm mainly related to birth trauma and leading to various degrees of weakness of the affected arm which may resolve during the first year of life
EUROCAT	European Surveillance of Congenital Anomalies
Fetal growth restriction	Evidence of abnormally slow growth of the fetus within the uterus; either estimated weight or abdominal circumference below the 10 th percentile, or slowing growth velocity of the abdominal circumference as measured at a subsequent ultrasound scan.
Fetal surveillance	The process of performing fetal well being tests (these may include ultrasound scans, fetal and placental Dopplers, biophysical profiles and fetal heart monitoring)
Folic acid	A water-soluble vitamin in the B-complex group which helps to prevent fetal neural tube defect when commenced by the mother before conception
Gestation	The time from conception to birth. The duration of gestation is measured from the first day of the last normal menstrual period
Gestational diabetes	Carbohydrate intolerance of varying severity which is diagnosed in pregnancy and resolves after pregnancy
Glucose electrode	Blood glucose measurement using electrochemical biosensors
Glycaemic control targets	Recommended levels of blood glucose
Glycaemic control test	A test that assesses how well blood glucose levels have been controlled over a period of time
Glycosylated haemoglobin	A test which measures the amount of glucose-bound haemoglobin and reflects how well the blood glucose level has been controlled over the previous 2 – 3 months
HbA1c	Glycosylated haemoglobin

High dependency care	Criteria for receipt of high-dependency care are:
	 • Receiving NCPAP for any part of the day but not fulfilling any of the criteria for intensive care
	 • Below 1000g current weight and not fulfilling any of the criteria for intensive care
	 • Receiving parenteral nutrition
	 • Having convulsions
	 • Receiving oxygen therapy and below 1500g current weight
	 • Requiring treatment for neonatal abstinence syndrome
	 • Requiring specific procedures that do not fulfil any criteria for intensive care:
	    • Care of intra-arterial catheter or chest drain
	    • Partial exchange transfusion
	    • Tracheostomy care until supervised by a parent
	    • Requiring frequent stimulation for severe apnoea.
	 (British Association of Perinatal Medicine, 2001)

Home blood glucose monitoring (HBGM)	Self-monitoring by the patient of blood glucose levels on a regular basis outside the hospital setting, using a blood glucose meter
Hyperplasia	An abnormal increase in the number of normal cells in normal arrangement in an organ or tissue, which increases its volume
Hypertension	High blood pressure
Hypoglycaemia	Low blood glucose level
Hypothermia	Abnormally low body temperature
Hypothyroidism	Deficiency of thyroid gland activity which leads to insufficient production of thyroid hormones
Induction of labour	The process of attempting to start labour (see spontaneous labour). A combination of pharmacological and physical methods may be used

Infant formula	An industrially produced milk product based on cow or soy milk, which aims to duplicate the nutrient content of natural human breast milk
Intensive care	Criteria for receipt of intensive care are: • Receiving any respiratory support via a tracheal tube and in the first 24 hours after its withdrawal • Receiving NCPAP for any part of the day and less than 5 days old • Below 1000g current weight and receiving NCPAP for any part of the day and for 24 hours after withdrawal • Less than 29 weeks of gestational age and less than 48 hours old • Requiring major emergency surgery, for the preoperative period and postoperatively for 24 hours • Requiring complex clinical procedures: 　• Full exchange transfusion 　• Peritoneal dialysis 　• Infusion of inotrope, pulmonary vasodilator or prostaglandin and for 24 hours afterwards. • Any other very unstable baby considered by the nurse-in-charge to need one-to-one nursing • A baby on the day of death. (British Association of Perinatal Medicine, 2001)
Interquartile range (IQR)	The spread of a set of values between which 25% (25th centile) and 75% (75th centile) of these values lie
Intrauterine death	Death of the fetus within the uterus before delivery
IUD	Intrauterine death
Late fetal loss	A death occurring between 20 weeks + 0 days and 23 weeks + 6 days
Late neonatal death	Death of a live born baby occurring from 7 completed days from the time of birth and before 28 completed days after birth.
Legal abortion	In England and Wales, term used to describe the deliberate ending of a pregnancy, under the provisions of the current law (1967/92 Act of Parliament), with the intention that the fetus will not survive
Macrosomia	Oversized baby as seen for example as a consequence of the effect of diabetes during pregnancy. Defined as having a birth weight above the 90th centile for gestation or a birth weight of 4000g or more.
Median	The value of the middle item of a series when the items are arranged in numerical order
Metformin	An oral antidiabetic agent that decreases glucose production by the liver and lowers plasma glucose levels
Microalbuminuria	A very small increase in urinary albumin
Miscarriage	Spontaneous ending of a pregnancy before viability (currently taken as 24 weeks of gestation)
MODY	Maturity onset diabetes of the young. A group of autosomal dominant disorders in young people each caused by a single gene defect, associated with decreased insulin production and varying degrees of clinical severity
Multidisciplinary clinic	A clinic with access to care from health professionals in more than one discipline. For diabetes, the disciplines recommended are obstetrics, diabetology, nursing, midwifery and dietetics.
Multiparous	A woman who has had at least one previous birth (from 24 weeks onwards)
Multiple birth	Birth of more than one baby from a pregnancy
Neonatal death	Death of a live born baby before 28 completed days after birth

Neonatal unit	A unit which provides additional care for babies over and above that which can be offered on a postnatal ward or transitional care unit. There are different levels of complexity of care which can be offered by an individual neonatal unit
Neural tube defect	A major birth defect caused by abnormal development of the neural tube, the structure present during embryonic life which later gives rise to the central nervous system (brain and spinal cord)
NHSLA	National Health Service Litigation Authority
NICE	National Institute for Health and Clinical Excellence
NSF	National Service Framework
Obesity	Increased body weight, defined as a Body Mass Index of 30 or greater
Odds ratio	A measure of the excess risk or degree of protection given by exposure to a certain factor. An odds ratio of greater than 1 shows an increased risk and less than 1 shows a protective effect
Offspring	Term encompassing live births, in utero losses after 20 completed weeks of gestation and terminations of pregnancy for congenital anomaly
Parity	The number of viable infants that a woman has delivered. Viability is currently accepted from 24 weeks of gestation onwards
Perinatal mortality rate	The number of stillbirths and early neonatal deaths per 1000 live and stillbirths
Placental insufficiency	Impairment of placental blood flow leading to impaired fetal growth and nutrition
Post-mortem examination	Examination of the body after death to determine cause of death
Postnatal	The period of time occurring after birth
Preconception care	Counselling and clinical management strategies before conception to ensure that women are well prepared for pregnancy. For women with diabetes, this includes ensuring near-normal glycaemic control before conception, commencing high dose folic acid, reviewing medication, screening for diabetes complications, and giving information about pregnancy risks, appropriate diet and lifestyle.
Preterm delivery	Delivery before 37+0 weeks' gestation
Preterm delivery rate	Percentage of all deliveries that occur before 37+0 weeks' gestation
Prevalence	The proportion of individuals in a population having a disease
Primary care	The health services that play a central role in the local community, such as general practitioners, health visitors, pharmacists, dentists and midwives
Primigravida	A woman who is in her first pregnancy
QDS	Quarter die sumendum (Latin) meaning four times a day
Quintile	The portion of a frequency distribution containing one fifth of the total sample
Range	The difference or interval between the smallest and largest values in a frequency distribution
Retinal assessment	Examining the fundi through pupils which have been dilated with eye drops
Secondary care	Services provided by medical specialists who generally do not have first contact with patients
Severe hypoglycaemia	Hypoglycaemia requiring help from another person
Shoulder dystocia	Any documented evidence of difficulty with delivering the shoulders after delivery of the baby's head
Singleton	One fetus or baby
Sliding scale	Intravenous insulin and dextrose infusions with a set of instructions for adjusting the dose of insulin on the basis of blood glucose test results

Stillbirth	Legal definition: a child that has issued forth from its mother after the 24th week of pregnancy and which did not at any time after being completely expelled from its mother breathe or show any other signs of life (Section 41 of the Births and Deaths Registration Act 1953 as amended by the Stillbirth Definition Act 1992)
Stillbirth rate	The number of stillbirths per 1000 total births (live births and stillbirths)
Termination of pregnancy	See Legal abortion
Thrombosis	The formation or presence of a clot of coagulated blood in a blood vessel
Thyroxine	An iodine-containing hormone produced by the thyroid gland
Transitional care unit	A unit providing care of term or near-term babies not needed high-dependency or intensive care, which can be safely delivered without babies being separated from their mothers
Trimester	One of the 3-month periods into which pregnancy is divided. The first trimester is 0-13 weeks of gestation, the second trimester is 14-26 weeks of gestation, and the third trimester is 27 weeks of gestation until birth.
Type 1 diabetes	There is an absolute deficiency of insulin production, due to autoimmune destruction of the insulin-producing beta cells in the islets of Langerhans in the pancreas. It accounts for 5 – 15% of all people with diabetes.
Type 2 diabetes	There is a relative deficiency of insulin production, and/or the insulin produced is not effective (insulin resistance). It accounts for 85% - 95% of all people with diabetes.
UK	United Kingdom
USS	Ultrasound scan

Foreword

This third and final report of the CEMACH national diabetes programme comes at an important time in the national drive to improve services for women with diabetes in pregnancy. The National Service Framework (NSF) for Diabetes requires the NHS to develop, implement and monitor policies that seek to empower and support women with diabetes to optimise the outcomes of their pregnancy. The CEMACH report shows that, whilst progress has been made in improving services for women with diabetes and their babies, there is much still to be done to meet the standards recommended by the NSF. Too many women continue to be poorly prepared for pregnancy in the critical areas of glycaemic control and folic acid supplementation. The report underlines the need for an increased focus on diabetes preconception care services and the development of strategies to educate women with diabetes of childbearing age. The growing proportion of women with type 2 diabetes during pregnancy, many of whom are from minority ethnic groups, presents an additional challenge for health services in developing responsive and accessible services.

This CEMACH report has identified several areas of good clinical practice during pregnancy in women with pre-existing diabetes. However, there continue to be areas where there is room for improvement, including antenatal fetal surveillance, glycaemic control during labour and delivery and postnatal diabetes care. The National Institute for Health and Clinical Excellence (NICE) is currently in the final stages of development of its new guideline for the management of diabetes in pregnancy. This guideline, when taken together with the CEMACH report, will provide local health services with an unprecedented wealth of material on which to base their development of improved services for women with diabetes in pregnancy.

Sir Liam Donaldson
Chief Medical Officer
Department of Health, England

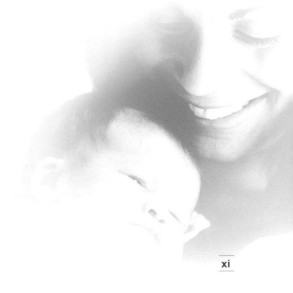

Preface

The Confidential Enquiry into Maternal and Child Health (CEMACH) is a unique study into diabetes and pregnancy which gives us a much needed insight into the issues surrounding this important time of a woman's life. Previous modules of CEMACH's diabetes programme have highlighted the increased risk of stillbirth, perinatal mortality and congenital anomaly for babies of women with diabetes. They also showed that women were often poorly prepared for pregnancy and that the care they received within the NHS was not always appropriate.

Now, the final enquiry module, which includes an audit of standards of care, has revealed a worrying lack of emphasis on care prior to pregnancy. The final report draws together a wealth of information and shows us the way forward by giving clear recommendations that will help improve the chances of women with diabetes to have a successful pregnancy.

It is crucial that women with diabetes are made fully aware of the risks they face before they become pregnant. Those looking after them then need to ensure that all the right steps are being taken to allow women to effectively reduce those risks. The fact that currently many women with diabetes enter pregnancy with poor glycaemic control is of great concern. Better care provision prior to pregnancy should help address the issue. The report also shows that social deprivation in women with diabetes is associated with poor pregnancy outcome. We now need to make sure that services are better targeted to reach the most vulnerable members of our communities.

At a time when the prevalence of both type 1 and type 2 diabetes in the UK is increasing rapidly, Diabetes UK believes that the recommendations made in the Confidential Enquiry into Maternal and Child Health's final diabetes in pregnancy report, need to be taken forward by health service professionals and commissioners alike.

Positive changes are needed to make sure that pregnancy and childbirth remain a time of hope and joy for women with diabetes.

Douglas Smallwood
Chief Executive
Diabetes UK

1. Introduction

This is the final report of the Confidential Enquiry into Maternal and Child Health (CEMACH) Diabetes Programme, which commenced in 2002. The programme has focused on pregnancy in women with type 1 and type 2 diabetes (with gestational diabetes excluded) and has included 3 modules:

1. A survey of diabetes maternity services for women with type 1 and type 2 diabetes in England, Wales and Northern Ireland.[1]
2. A descriptive study of 3808 pregnancies to women with type 1 and type 2 diabetes in England, Wales and Northern Ireland who were identified at any time between booking and delivery from 1 March 2002 to 28 February 2003, with follow up to pregnancy outcome at 28 days after delivery.[2]
3. A national confidential enquiry reviewing demographic, social and lifestyle factors, and clinical care in 442 pregnancies to women with type 1 and type 2 diabetes, and their association with pregnancy outcomes. The results of this last module are included within this report.

1.1 Context of the CEMACH Diabetes Programme

The topic of diabetes and pregnancy was chosen by CEMACH for a number of reasons:

- Diabetes is a common medical disorder complicating pregnancy, affecting 1 in 250 women in England, Wales and Northern Ireland.
- In the mid-1990s, women with diabetes continued to have an increased risk of perinatal mortality, stillbirth and poor pregnancy outcomes compared to the general maternity population[3-5] despite the St. Vincent's Declaration in 1989[6], which set a 5 year target for women with diabetes to achieve similar pregnancy outcomes to women without diabetes.
- In 2001, the Diabetes National Service Framework (NSF)[7], set out national standards for the management of diabetes and pregnancy. The CEMACH Diabetes Programme offered the opportunity to provide a national overview of maternity service provision and clinical care for women with diabetes, which could be used to evaluate progress in implementation of the NSF.

1.2 Aims of the national enquiry

The aims of the enquiry module were:

- To investigate standards of care provided to women with type 1 and type 2 diabetes in England, Wales and Northern Ireland and identify any underlying issues.
- To investigate any associations between poor pregnancy outcomes and demographic, social and lifestyle, and clinical care factors.
- To investigate any associations between demographic and clinical characteristics, social and lifestyle factors, and clinical care with type of diabetes.

1.3 A need for change

The prevalence of diabetes in the general population is increasing rapidly, due partly to an increasing contribution from particular ethnic minority groups, and increasing obesity in the general population. Type 2 diabetes is being diagnosed more frequently in younger age groups including children.[8] This is likely to result in a continuing increase in the numbers of women with diabetes of childbearing age in

England, Wales and Northern Ireland, which has significant implications for both primary and secondary care health services.

The National Institute for Health and Clinical Excellence (NICE) is due to publish a national guideline on diabetes in pregnancy in November 2007, and this is anticipated to provide health professionals with guidance on best practice supported by current evidence.

CEMACH's findings will contribute to the evidence-base for this guideline, and it is hoped that the findings and recommendations of this report will also help the NHS to identify any gaps in current services and work towards improving care and ultimately outcomes for all women with type 1 and type 2 diabetes.

References

1. *Confidential Enquiry into Maternal and Child Health: Maternity services in 2002 for women with type 1 and type 2 diabetes, England, Wales and Northern Ireland.* CEMACH: London; 2004.
2. *Confidential Enquiry into Maternal and Child Health: Pregnancy in women with type 1 and type 2 diabetes in 2002-03, England, Wales and Northern Ireland.* CEMACH: London; 2005.
3. Casson IF, Clarke CA, Howard CV, McKendrick O, Pennycook S, Pharoah PO et al. *Outcomes of pregnancy in insulin dependent women with diabetes: results of a five year population cohort study.* BMJ 1997;315:275-82.
4. Hawthorne G, Robson S, Ryall EA, Sen D, Roberts SH, Ward Platt MP. *Prospective population based survey of outcome of pregnancy in women with diabetes: results of the Northern Diabetic Pregnancy Audit, 1994.* BMJ 1997; 315:279-81.
5. Hadden DR, Alexander A, McCance DR, Traub AI. *Obstetric and diabetic care for pregnancy in diabetic women: 10 years outcome analysis, 1985-1995.* Northern Ireland Diabetes Group, Ulster Obstetrical Society. Diabetic Med: 2001; 18:546-53.
6. *Workshop Report. Diabetes Care and Research in Europe: The Saint Vincent Declaration.* Diabetic Med: 1990; 7:360.
7. *National Service Framework for Diabetes (England) Standards.* Department of Health. The Stationery Office: London; 2001.
8. Ehtisham S. *The emergence of type 2 diabetes in childhood.* Annals of Clinical Biochemistry 41(Pt1): Jan 2004; 10-6.

2. Key findings of the CEMACH Diabetes Programme

The three modules of the CEMACH Diabetes Programme (the CEMACH survey of diabetes maternity services, the descriptive study of 3808 pregnancies to women with type 1 and type 2 diabetes, and the national enquiry into 521 diabetic pregnancies), have identified a number of key findings. These findings are summarised in this chapter. Additional details can be found in the two previous reports of the Diabetes Programme and in the relevant chapters of this report.

2.1 Social and demographic characteristics

Women with type 1 diabetes accounted for 73% (2767/3808) of women in the descriptive study and women with type 2 diabetes accounted for 27% (1041/3808) of women in the descriptive study.[1]

Women with type 2 diabetes were more likely to be older, multiparous, live in a deprived area and come from a Black, Asian or Other Ethnic minority group, than women with type 1 diabetes.[1]

In the enquiry, maternal social deprivation (based on postcode of residence) was associated with poor pregnancy outcome.

Smoking before pregnancy in women with diabetes was associated with an increased risk of poor pregnancy outcome. Further work is required to elucidate the interrelationship and relative contribution of factors such as smoking, deprivation and ethnicity to pregnancy outcome in women with diabetes.

2.2 Clinical characteristics

In the descriptive study, there was a 36% preterm delivery rate and a 67% caesarean section rate for women with diabetes.[1] This compares to a 7% preterm delivery rate and a 22% caesarean section rate in the general maternity population.[2]

In the descriptive study, 21% of singleton babies of women with diabetes had a birth weight of 4000g or more compared to 11% of singleton babies in the general maternity population in England, 2002-03.[1] 8% of babies in the descriptive study had shoulder dystocia, compared with 3% in a regional general maternity population.[3]

There was a ten-fold increased incidence of Erb's palsy in babies of women with diabetes compared to babies in the general maternity population in the UK.[1, 4]

Nearly half of women in the enquiry had recurrent hypoglycaemia during pregnancy and more than a tenth had at least one severe hypoglycaemic episode requiring external help. There was no evidence from case-control analysis that hypoglycaemia was associated with a poor pregnancy outcome for the baby.

2.3 Pregnancy outcomes

In the descriptive study, women with diabetes had significantly increased risks of adverse pregnancy outcome compared to the general maternity population: a fivefold increased risk of stillbirth, a threefold increased risk of perinatal mortality and a twofold increased risk of fetal congenital anomaly.[1]

A number of demographic and clinical characteristics, social and lifestyle factors, and clinical care factors were associated with poor pregnancy outcome, and are discussed in detail in other chapters of this report.

2.4 Preconception care

In the CEMACH survey of maternity services, less than a fifth of maternity units in England, Wales and Northern Ireland provided structured multidisciplinary preconception care for women with diabetes.[5]

Women with diabetes were poorly prepared for pregnancy:

- Less than half were recorded to take folic acid supplements prior to pregnancy
- Less than half were recorded to have had preconception counselling regarding glycaemic control, diet, contraception, diabetes complications and alcohol intake
- A third were recorded to have a test of glycaemic control in the 6 months before pregnancy[1]
- Two-thirds had evidence of suboptimal glycaemic control before conception and in the first trimester of pregnancy.

Suboptimal preconception care, glycaemic control before and during pregnancy and approach of the woman to managing her diabetes were all associated with poor pregnancy outcome.

One of the main underlying factors to suboptimal preconception care was failure of provision of appropriate care by health professionals: preconception counselling, contraceptive advice, provision of high dose folic acid, and appropriate screening and management of diabetes complications.

The main factors underlying suboptimal glycaemic control and a suboptimal approach to managing diabetes were social and lifestyle issues: non-attendance of women at planned appointments, non-adherence to medical advice about diabetes management, unplanned pregnancy and social factors including language difficulties, difficult domestic circumstances and erratic or busy lifestyles.

Only a minority of women in the enquiry appeared to be using any form of contraception in the 12 months before pregnancy, based on documentation by adult diabetes services and primary care. This suggests that women are not aware of the importance of continuing effective contraception until their glycaemic control is as near-normal as possible.

In the enquiry, a minority of women were documented to be on high dose (5mg) folic acid before pregnancy.

There was poor documentation of preconception care and advice given.

2.5 Clinical care during pregnancy

Suboptimal maternity care during pregnancy was associated with poor pregnancy outcome. Underlying issues identified included suboptimal fetal surveillance (both cardiotocograph and ultrasound monitoring) and poor management of maternal risks identified during the course of pregnancy.

Suboptimal diabetes care (excluding glycaemic control) during pregnancy was associated with poor pregnancy outcome.

Suboptimal fetal surveillance of babies with antenatal evidence of macrosomia (defined for the enquiry as evidence of fetal size greater than the 90th centile for gestation) was associated with poor pregnancy outcome. The main underlying issues identified were lack of timely follow up and poor interpretation of ultrasound scans.

2.6 Differences between women with type 1 and type 2 diabetes

In the enquiry, women with type 2 diabetes were more likely to be obese than women with type 1 diabetes.

In the 12 months prior to pregnancy, women with type 2 diabetes were less likely than women with type 1 diabetes to have a retinal assessment, a test for albuminuria and to be recorded to be using contraception.

Women with type 1 diabetes were more likely than women with type 2 diabetes to have recurrent hypoglycaemia during pregnancy or episodes of hypoglycaemia requiring external help. Nevertheless, a fifth of pregnant women with type 2 diabetes had recurrent hypoglycaemia.

Fewer women with type 2 diabetes than type 1 diabetes had a retinal assessment in the first trimester of pregnancy (or at booking if later).

2.7 Clinical governance issues

In the CEMACH survey of maternity services[5], nearly two-thirds of maternity units in England, Wales and Northern Ireland self-reported a multidisciplinary antenatal team that included all the health professionals (obstetrician, diabetes physician, midwife, diabetes specialist nurse, dietitian) recommended by the Diabetes National Service Framework.[6]

There was poor documentation of both obstetric and diabetes care for more than half of women in the enquiry.

Concerns were raised at panel enquiry about the standard of local guidelines for three-quarters of women in the enquiry.

2.8 Neonatal care of term babies of women with diabetes

In the CEMACH survey carried out in 2002-03[5], nearly a third of units had a policy of routinely admitting babies of mothers with diabetes to the neonatal unit.

In the neonatal enquiry (see Chapter 12, Neonatal care of women with diabetes), one third of term babies were admitted to a neonatal unit for special care and over half of these admissions were avoidable.

Intention to breastfeed was lower among mothers with diabetes than the breastfeeding rate in the general population.[1] There appeared to be several barriers to breastfeeding, including maternal choice, infant formula given despite maternal choice to breastfeed, and some babies not receiving an early feed soon after birth.

Blood glucose testing of the baby was being carried out too early following delivery, and inappropriate methods of testing were often used.

Two thirds of babies in the neonatal enquiry had suboptimal care on the labour ward and this frequently impacted on subsequent care.

2.9 Postnatal care

Half of women in the enquiry had suboptimal postnatal diabetes care. The main underlying issues were poor management of glycaemic control after delivery, lack of contact with the diabetes team, inadequate plans of care at discharge from hospital, and no contraceptive advice given to women.

Women who had a poor pregnancy outcome were more likely not to receive postnatal contraceptive advice and were more likely to have had suboptimal postnatal diabetes care.

In the enquiry, women with type 2 diabetes were less likely to receive postnatal contraceptive advice.

References

1. *Confidential Enquiry into Maternal and Child Health. Pregnancy in women with type 1 and type 2 diabetes in 2002-03, England, Wales and Northern Ireland.* CEMACH: London; 2005.
2. *The National Sentinel Caesarean Section Audit Report.* Royal College of Obstetricians and Gynaecologists, Clinical Effectiveness Support Unit. RCOG Press: London; 2001.
3. Nesbitt TS, Gilbert WM, Herrhen B. *Shoulder dystocia and associated risk factors with macrosomic infants born in California.* Am J Obstet Gynecol; Aug 1998; 179:476-80.
4. Evans-Jones G, Kay SP, Weindling AM, Cranny G, Ward A, Bradshaw A, et al. *Congenital brachial palsy: incidence, causes, and outcomes in the United Kingdom and Republic of Ireland.* Arch Dis Child Fetal Neonatal Ed; 2003; 88:F185-9.
5. *Confidential Enquiry into Maternal and Child Health. Maternity services in 2002 for women with type 1 and type 2 diabetes, England, Wales and Northern Ireland.* CEMACH: London; 2004.
6. *National Service Framework for Diabetes (England) Standards.* Department of Health. The Stationery Office: London; 2001.

3. Summary of recommendations

This chapter includes the recommendations that have been made arising from the findings of this report. Details of the process followed to derive the recommendations can be found in Chapter 5.

The recommendations below apply to all women with type 1 and type 2 diabetes.

Social and lifestyle issues

Clinical

1. Preconception and maternity services related to pregnancy should be easily accessible and responsive to all women with diabetes, and provide appropriate care and information.
2. There should be mechanisms in place to identify vulnerable communities and individuals, so that additional services can be provided as appropriate to women of childbearing age with diabetes, thereby ensuring optimal preconception care.
3. Providers of diabetes care should develop educational strategies that will enable all women of childbearing age with diabetes to prepare adequately for pregnancy.

Audit and research

4. Research should be carried out to:
   - identify the barriers to accessing preconception care
   - identify possible strategies to support self-care and pregnancy planning by women with diabetes.

Clinical issues: preconception

Clinical

1. Commissioners of services must ensure that all women with diabetes are provided with specialist preconception services, with access to all members of the specialist multidisciplinary team.
   As a minimum, these services should include:
   - Clear signposting to different aspects of care
   - Diet and lifestyle advice
   - Provision of appropriate contraception
   - Higher dose folic acid supplementation
   - Smoking cessation support
   - Assessment and management of diabetes complications
   - Setting of glycaemic control targets and regular discussion of results of self-monitoring, to enable the woman to achieve control that is as near to normal as possible before conception
   - Discussion of diabetes pregnancy risks and expected management strategies
   - Clear documentation of care and counselling, ideally using a standard template.

Audit and research

2. Preconception services should be audited to ensure that minimum standards are being met.

Clinical issues: pregnancy

Clinical

1. An individualised care plan covering the pregnancy and postnatal period up to 6 weeks should be clearly documented in the notes, ideally using a standard template. The plan may require changes to be made depending on the clinical circumstances through pregnancy. As a minimum, the care plan should include:
   - Targets for glycaemic control
   - Retinal screening schedule
   - Renal screening schedule
   - Fetal surveillance
   - Plan for delivery
   - Diabetes care after delivery.
2. The care plan should be implemented from the outset of pregnancy by a multidisciplinary team present at the same time in the same clinic. As a minimum, the multidisciplinary team should include an obstetrician, diabetes physician, diabetes specialist nurse, diabetes midwife and dietitian.
3. Pregnancies with ultrasound evidence of macrosomia should have a clear management plan put in place by a consultant obstetrician. This should include timing of follow-up scans, fetal surveillance and mode and timing of delivery.
4. A care plan for postnatal management should be clearly documented in the notes for all women. As a minimum, this should include:
   - Plan for management of glycaemic control
   - Neonatal care
   - Contraception
   - Follow-up care after discharge from hospital.

Audit and research

5. Research should be carried out to investigate:
   - the most appropriate management strategy following antenatal evidence of macrosomia in babies of women with diabetes
   - how best to achieve optimal blood glucose control during pregnancy, labour and delivery.

Clinical governance

Clinical

1. Commissioners should recognise the complexity of diabetes management immediately before and during pregnancy, and ensure that the available service provision includes all members of the multidisciplinary team.

2. Patient pathways of care including preconception counselling, pregnancy care and post-pregnancy management should be incorporated into the clinical record.
3. Services should review their local guidelines. The NICE Diabetes in Pregnancy guideline, due to be published in November 2007, is anticipated to provide current evidence for best practice.
4. In order to raise awareness, specialist multidisciplinary teams should provide regular educational days for all primary and secondary care professionals likely to be involved in the care of women with diabetes in the local population, to cover all aspects of preconception, pregnancy and postnatal care.

Audit and research

5. Diabetes networks should carry out regular audits of preconception and pregnancy services.

Type 1 and type 2 diabetes

Clinical

1. During pregnancy, retinal and renal screening schedules should be provided for both women with type 1 and women with type 2 diabetes.
2. Advice about hypoglycaemia during pregnancy, including prevention and management strategies, should be provided to both women with type 1 diabetes and women with type 2 diabetes.

Audit and research

3. Diabetes networks should audit standards of preconception and pregnancy care for both women with type 1 and women with type 2 diabetes.

Neonatal care of term babies of women with diabetes

1. All units delivering women with diabetes should have a written policy for the management of the baby. The policy should assume that babies will remain with their mothers in the absence of complications.
2. Mothers with diabetes should be informed antenatally of the beneficial effects of breastfeeding on metabolic control for both themselves, and their babies.
3. Mothers with diabetes should be offered an opportunity for skin-to-skin contact with their babies immediately after delivery. Breastfeeding within one hour of birth should be encouraged.
4. Blood glucose testing performed too early should be avoided in well babies, without signs of hypoglycaemia. Testing should be performed before a feed, using a reliable method (ward-based glucose electrode or laboratory analysis). For all blood glucose tests, the time it is performed, method used, result, and action taken should be clearly documented in the notes. Further research is needed to define the optimal timing of first blood glucose test in babies of diabetic mothers.
5. Junior paediatric staff should be trained in the management of babies of mothers with diabetes. This should include appreciation of the importance of supporting early breastfeeding, avoidance of early blood glucose testing in the well baby, and formulation of a written plan agreed with the mother.
6. Midwives should recognise the importance of supporting early breastfeeding for women with diabetes, and the need to document this aspect of care.

4. Methodology

4.1 Introduction

The enquiry module of the CEMACH diabetes programme encompassed a case-control study, a comparison of type 1 and type 2 diabetes, and an audit of care:

- A case-control analysis to examine any differences in demographic factors, social and lifestyle issues, and clinical care between a) pregnancies resulting in adverse pregnancy outcome (deaths from 20 weeks gestation up to 28 days after delivery or major fetal congenital anomaly at any gestation) and b) pregnancies resulting in a normally formed baby surviving to 28 days of life.
- A comparison of any differences in demographic factors, social and lifestyle issues, and clinical care between women with a) type 1 and b) type 2 diabetes.
- An audit of the care received before, during and after pregnancy by a subset of women within the whole study population of the CEMACH diabetes programme.

4.2 Selection of pregnancies for enquiry

To enable the audit of care and case-control analysis to be conducted, four groups of pregnancies were selected for enquiry:

1. **Anomalies** – pregnancy to a woman with type 1 or type 2 diabetes resulting in a singleton baby (including terminations of pregnancy at any gestation, late fetal losses, stillbirths and live births) with a confirmed major congenital anomaly, diagnosed up to 28 days of life.
2. **Deaths** – pregnancy to a woman with type 1 or type 2 diabetes resulting in death of a singleton baby from 20 weeks of gestation up to 28 days after delivery, excluding terminations of pregnancy and confirmed congenital anomalies.
3. **Controls** – pregnancy to a woman with type 1 or type 2 diabetes resulting in a singleton birth delivering at 20 weeks of gestation onwards and surviving to 28 days of life, excluding those with a confirmed congenital anomaly.

Preliminary findings from the CEMACH descriptive study of 3808 pregnancies to women with diabetes in England, Wales and Northern Ireland in 2002-03 showed that women with type 2 diabetes appeared to be more poorly prepared for pregnancy and also had an equivalent risk of adverse pregnancy outcome to women with type 1 diabetes.[1,2] It was therefore decided to enquire on an additional sample of pregnancies of women with type 2 diabetes to enable a more thorough investigation of the care received by these women.

4. **Additional type 2 sample** – pregnancy to a woman with type 2 diabetes resulting in a singleton birth delivering at 20 weeks of gestation onwards and surviving to 28 days of life, excluding those with a confirmed congenital anomaly.

All pregnancies meeting the definition of anomaly or death within the CEMACH descriptive study were selected to form the cases for the case-control analysis. Controls were randomly sampled from the group of pregnancies reported in the CEMACH descriptive study fitting the definition of a control in order to sample one control per case. The additional type 2 pregnancies were randomly sampled from the pregnancies meeting this definition (see 4. above) after exclusion of the type 2 pregnancies which had already been sampled as controls.

All the chapters in this report apart from Chapters 5, 10, 11 and 12 refer to the cases and controls described above.

The additional sample of type 2 pregnancies was used only in the analysis examining differences between women with type 1 and type 2 diabetes, and the methodology for this analysis is described separately in Chapter 11.

In total, 590 pregnancies were sampled for enquiry. Notes were requested from the unit of delivery and followed up on three occasions over the subsequent three months. Notes were unable to be retrieved for 12% of all notes requested giving a final total of 521 pregnancies going for enquiry (table 4.1).

Table 4.1			
Summary of notes requested and received			
Type of pregnancy	Total requested	Notes not available	Notes received
Control	245	25	220
Death	110	15	95
Anomaly	138	11	127
Additional Type 2	97	18	79
Total	590	69	521

4.3 Panel process

Medical records of all pregnancies in the enquiry module were reviewed by multidisciplinary enquiry panels of senior health care professionals, held at regional level. Panels reviewed three or four cases per meeting. Cases reviewed were selected from a national pool excluding the region of the assessing panel, to ensure an independent assessment of the care provided.

In total, 143 panel meetings were convened between April 2004 and December 2005 in the CEMACH regions throughout England, Wales and Northern Ireland. Panel meetings did not take place in the West Midlands region but any pregnancy to a woman delivering in the West Midlands that was selected for enquiry was included in the national pool and reviewed by enquiry panels outside of the West Midlands.

4.3.1 Panel chairs

Two or three panel chairs were appointed per region by a central selection committee. The specific remit of the panel chairs was to ensure that an equitable process was followed to reach consensus on each of the specific questions asked in the enquiry pro forma. Panel chairs were invited to attend a training day before the commencement of the panel process. This allowed an opportunity to discuss various challenges likely to be faced by a panel chair and to develop mechanisms of working that would ensure a consistent approach to panel enquiry meetings across the regions.

4.3.2 Panel composition

Each panel for the diabetes enquiry consisted of two of each of the following disciplines:

- Obstetrician
- Midwife
- Diabetes specialist nurse
- Diabetes physician.

At least one clinician from each specialty was required to be present in order for the panel meeting to take place. Under exceptional circumstances the panel chair could participate as a full assessor if there were no other clinicians available from their specific discipline. If it was not possible for at least one clinician from each specialty to be represented then the panel meeting was cancelled. Additional panel members whose input was relevant to particular enquiry cases were invited to attend meetings as required e.g. general practitioners, pathologists, neonatologists.

Previous confidential enquiries had not included lay panel assessors. For the diabetes enquiry, CEMACH sought to include lay assessors on the enquiry panels. Criteria for lay panel assessors were agreed with Diabetes UK, and the initiative was piloted in 2 regions. One lay member attended 5 panel meetings in Yorkshire and Humberside region.

Observers were allowed to attend (with due notice) but were not expected to contribute to the discussion during assessment.

In total, 647 health professionals contributed over 5000 hours to panel enquiries over the course of the enquiry module, with 70 additional observers attending one or more panels. The median number of cases reviewed by each assessor was 8 (range 4-48).

4.4 Enquiry documentation

Panel members were provided with the medical records for each case pertaining to care in the antenatal, delivery and postnatal periods. These included diabetes and maternity notes plus any relevant drug charts, haematology, biochemistry and histology results. Neonatal notes up to day 3 post delivery were also provided where applicable. Following a feasibility exercise at the outset of the project it was deemed impractical to collect all medical records pertaining to diabetes care prior to the pregnancy of interest. In order to allow some assessment of care in the pre-pregnancy period a pre-pregnancy pro forma was also completed by a health professional involved in the preconception care of the woman, either within the adult diabetes service or in primary care (see Appendix A). In addition, any professional correspondence relating to diabetes management within the year preceding the last menstrual period was requested. Women were not contacted directly at any stage of this process, and information about social and lifestyle issues and clinical care was therefore based solely on documentation provided by the health professionals involved in the care of the woman and her baby.

In order to maintain confidentiality of the women, their families and the health professionals involved in their care, all notes provided to panel assessors were anonymised by the CEMACH regional managers in order to remove any identifiable information. This included patient identifiers, hospital identifiers and staff identifiers. Where names of staff were anonymised, the designation (grade) of the staff member was entered onto the documentation, to enable panel assessment of whether care had been provided by the appropriate grade of staff.

4.5 Assessment of care

The scope of this enquiry included preconception care, care during pregnancy, labour and delivery, and postnatal and neonatal care up to 3 days post delivery. A structured enquiry pro forma (see Appendix B) was developed by the CEMACH central office with advice from members of the CEMACH Diabetes Professional Advisory Group. This pro forma contained a mixture of factual questions and assessments of care from review of the medical records, after a round-table discussion and after panel consensus had been reached. Panel assessors were asked to grade their opinion of the quality of care as 'optimal', 'adequate' or 'poor'. 'Optimal' indicated that there were no issues with care, while 'adequate' indicated that there were some issues of concern. 'Adequate' and 'poor' care were aggregated as 'suboptimal' care for the purpose of analysis.

If concerns had been identified, panels were asked to describe the key issues contributing to this assessment and to code the issues according to the following categories:

Issues relating directly to the patient and/or family issues	
PD	Duration or severity of diabetes.
PO	Other complicating medical or social and / or lifestyle factors which may hinder optimal management e.g. management-intensive medical conditions such as thrombophilia or cardiac disease, and social factors such as housing problems or lack of family support.
PC	Woman actively chose not to follow the medical advice given e.g. refusal to undergo induction of labour until 42+ weeks of gestation.
PA	Woman's actions detracted from optimal management e.g. infrequent home blood glucose monitoring, not following dietary instructions.
PN	Woman did not attend appointments e.g. failure to attend for clinic visits or ultrasound scans.

Issues relating to the provision of health services	
HP	Clinical practice e.g. no timely discussion of timing and mode of delivery.
HC	Communication. This could be a failure of communication between professionals caring for the woman e.g. inadequate discussion between obstetrician and physician, or a failure of communication between professionals and the woman e.g. interpreting services were not adequate despite difficulties with English.
HR	Resources including staffing e.g. no dietitian in the antenatal clinic, lack of midwifery staff on labour ward, problems with accessing timely fetal surveillance such as growth scans.

Panels were asked to code up to four issues that were appropriate to the judgment of 'adequate' or 'poor' care. During analysis, these codes were used as a guide for the analysis of the themes arising from the free text.

4.5.1 Panel guidance

Some questions in the enquiry pro forma included guidance for the panel assessors. The purpose of this guidance was to aid consistent definitions but was not prescriptive, recognising that panel assessors may have had access to information at panel enquiry which was at variance with the guidance provided.

4.6 Case-control analysis

For the purposes of the case-control analysis, four distinct sets of analyses were performed. The following four groups were classed as cases and compared with all controls

1. Anomalies, as per definition above (Figure 4.1, B+C)
2. Deaths excluding anomalies, as per definition above (Figure 4.1, A only)
3. All deaths, including deaths with congenital anomaly (Figure 4.1, A+B)
4. Poor pregnancy outcome - all adverse outcomes formed by groups 1 and 2 together (Figure 4.1, A+B+C)

Figure 4.1
Selection of cases for case-control analysis

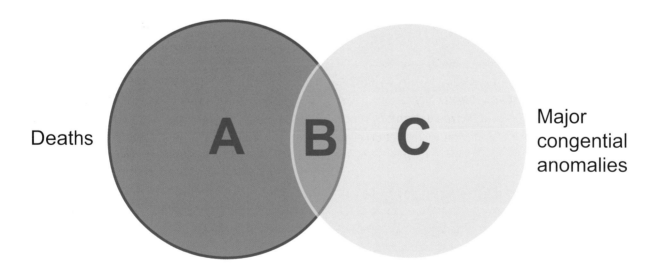

Deaths — A B C — Major congential anomalies

Associations in the main body of the report are those for group 4 i.e. poor pregnancy outcome. Results from the additional analyses are included in Appendices C, D and E. Analyses are reported as odds ratios examining the association between each factor of interest and adverse pregnancy outcome compared to the control group. Adjusted odds ratios are presented where appropriate. Where there are notable differences between any of the four case definitions in the direction and/or magnitude of a particular association, these are referenced in the text.

When deriving odds ratios for any particular factor, information for any particular question which was recorded as 'not documented' or 'missing', were excluded from the analysis. However, when documented evidence of care was investigated (in Chapters 7 – 9), 'not documented' was included in the analysis.

4.7 Type 1 versus type 2 analysis

The methodology for this analysis is described in Chapter 11.

4.8 Analysis of panel comments

Panel assessment of the quality of care before, during and after pregnancy was assessed as optimal versus suboptimal, where suboptimal reflected a combination of 'adequate' (some issues with care) and 'poor' responses.

Where a case was considered to have had suboptimal care, panels were asked to summarise the key issues (see enquiry assessment above). These free text fields were categorised into one or more theme headings by an individual clinician (obstetrician, diabetes physician or neonatologist as appropriate) to allow further exploration of the data. Tables where free text information has been categorised are footnoted throughout the report. Categorisation was based purely on the text contained in the pro forma.

4.9 Derivation of recommendations

Recommendations were derived following consultation with all members of the CEMACH Diabetes Professional Advisory Group (PAG) and with regional panel chairs. The draft report was reviewed by the Diabetes PAG and suggested recommendations sent by individual PAG members to the CEMACH central office. These recommendations were collated and sent to all PAG members for scoring. Suggested recommendations were scored for validity (whether the recommendation was based on the findings of the report) on a scale of 1-4, where 1 was extremely valid and 4 was not at all valid; and for clinical importance (the potential of the recommendation to impact on clinical practice or outcomes) on a scale of 1-4, where 1 was of high clinical importance and 4 was of no clinical importance.

Any individual recommendation with a median score of 4 for validity **or** clinical importance was excluded. The scored recommendations were then sent out for consultation to regional panel chairs for a second round of scoring. Panel chairs were also invited to make any additional recommendations they felt were both valid and clinically important.

Following a second round of scoring and analysis, a meeting of the Diabetes PAG and regional panel chairs was held to review all scored recommendations and reach consensus on inclusion of recommendations within the report. These revised recommendations were collated and reviewed by the Chair of the Diabetes PAG and CEMACH Central Office, and recommendations then sent out again to PAG members and panel chairs for comments. Comments received were reviewed, final revisions made, and the recommendations then finalised by CEMACH Central Office.

4.10 Limitations

All data collected during this enquiry were derived from review of the medical records. Findings of this report are therefore based on documentation in the medical records of demographic factors, social and lifestyle issues and clinical care, and are not based on direct questioning of clinicians or women.

In many cases it was not possible to complete all questions on the pro forma with reference to the medical notes provided. The proportion of missing information was even more pronounced for information pertaining to the pre-pregnancy period, where missing data ranged from less than 5% to more than 50% for specific data items.

Throughout the report, numbers are reported with reference to the total number of records where information was recorded i.e. excluding all missing data. In general, there was no systematic difference in the number of missing responses dependent on whether a pregnancy was a case or a control.

With regard to panel assessment of women's behaviour and clinical care, it should be noted that the enquiry sample is not fully representative of the whole population of pregnant women with diabetes, as approximately half of women in the enquiry had a poor pregnancy outcome due to the sampling process. It is therefore possible that the issues identified by enquiry panels represent the worse end of the spectrum of suboptimal behaviour and care. However, for many factors examined there was no difference between cases and controls.

One of the potential limitations to the panel enquiry approach is variation of assessments between different regional panels. Panel guidance notes were provided in order to minimise variation, and the panel chairs and regional managers had an important role to play in directing the discussion and ensuring that all factors were taken into consideration during assessments. Panel chairs attended a training day (as described above) in order to standardise the approach to the enquiry assessment, and guidance was provided in the enquiry pro forma (see appendix B) to aid in its completion. Despite this training and guidance there remains a degree of subjectivity in the panel assessment process which cannot be completely eliminated.

A source of bias that has been previously experienced in some confidential enquiry programmes is that knowledge of the pregnancy outcome may affect the panel assessment of care. The Project 27/28 study[3] which enquired into standards of care for babies born at 27 and 28 weeks gestation, blinded assessors to the outcome of the case up to the point of delivery. In this study, as one of the outcomes was congenital anomaly which could be diagnosed antenatally, it was not possible to blind the panels to pregnancy outcome in all cases. For this reason, it was agreed that assessors would not be blinded to any outcomes for the pregnancies being reviewed. This may have led to an element of bias in this study particularly with respect to the questions which asked for panel assessment of the standard of care received or the woman's approach to managing her diabetes. This bias could have led to an overestimate of the extent of the association of panel assessment of suboptimal care with adverse pregnancy outcome. Results relating to panel assessment are clearly identified throughout the report and should be interpreted with a degree of caution.

Associations are reported in Chapters 6–10 for poor pregnancy outcome, which combines two separate adverse outcomes, fetal congenital anomaly and death from 20 weeks of gestation, compared to controls. In some cases, this precludes a more specific focus on the impact of the particular behaviour or care factor on individual poor outcomes e.g. fetal anomalies. For this reason, Appendices C, D, and E have been included to provide information on associations with poor outcome for each additional case definition (fetal congenital anomalies, all deaths, and deaths excluding anomalies).

It is recognised that some of the factors reported to have an association with adverse outcome are not likely to be on the causal pathway, for example poor glycaemic control after the first trimester of pregnancy is unlikely to have been causative for fetal congenital anomaly, and poor diabetes care after delivery is not causative for poor pregnancy outcome. However, there may be other explanations for these associations, and they have therefore been retained, with discussion in the text where appropriate.

Results reported within chapter 6 are crude odds ratios examining each potential risk factor or assessment of clinical care and its association with poor pregnancy outcome in isolation. In order to allow for potential confounding factors, all odds ratios were adjusted for the effect of maternal age and deprivation on pregnancy outcome and these are also displayed. These adjusted odds ratios are displayed throughout chapters 7-9. It is possible, however, that there are additional confounding factors or interactions which have not been allowed for in this analysis.

1.11 The diabetes neonatal enquiry

Details on the methodology and derivation of recommendations for the diabetes neonatal enquiry can be found in Chapter 12.

References

1. *Confidential Enquiry into Maternal and Child Health: Pregnancy in women with type 1 and type 2 diabetes in 2002-03, England, Wales and Northern Ireland*. CEMACH: London; 2005.
2. Macintosh M, Fleming K, Bailey J, Doyle P, Modder J, Acolet D, et al. *Perinatal mortality and congenital anomalies in babies of women with type 1 or type 2 diabetes in England, Wales and Northern Ireland: population based study*. BMJ, Jul 22 2006 333 (7560):177.
3. *Confidential Enquiry into Stillbirths and Deaths in Infancy. Project 27/28: An Enquiry into quality of care and its effect on the survival of babies born at 27-28 weeks*. The Stationery Office: London; 2003.

5. A description of women and babies in the enquiry

5.1 Introduction

This chapter describes the 442 women and 442 offspring in the enquiry module of the CEMACH Diabetes Programme, after excluding the additional 79 pregnant women with type 2 diabetes sampled for the purpose of carrying out a comparison between type 1 and type 2 diabetes (see Chapters 4 and 11).

Multiple births were excluded before sampling from the 3808 pregnancies in the descriptive study (see Chapter 4 for details of sampling methods). All babies who died from 20 weeks gestation up to 28 days after delivery, and all fetal congenital anomalies, were sampled for enquiry, together with a random sample of controls (singleton babies without a congenital anomaly surviving to day 28) so that there was one control for each case sampled. Women with poor pregnancy outcomes therefore represented a higher proportion of the enquiry sample than of the 3808 pregnancies in the descriptive study (approximately 50% of pregnancies in the enquiry module versus less than 10% of all pregnancies in the descriptive study).[1]

5.2 The women

5.2.1 Socio-demographic characteristics

The women in the enquiry were very similar to the whole population sampled from with respect to socio-demographic characteristics (table 5.1). Slightly more women in the enquiry were in the more deprived quintiles compared to women in the descriptive study.

5.2.2 Diabetes complications

Twelve percent of 359 women in the enquiry had nephropathy (panel guidance was that this could be incipient with microalbuminuria or established with persistent dipstick positive proteinuria and/or serum creatinine greater than 130mmol/l).

Thirty two percent of 316 women had retinopathy (pre-existing or diagnosed for the first time in pregnancy) (table 5.2). Fifty one percent of 400 women in the enquiry had recurrent hypoglycaemia during pregnancy and 20% of 311 women had at least one severe hypoglycaemic episode requiring external help.

Information on specific diabetes complications was not collected for the descriptive study of 3808 pregnancies so direct comparisons cannot be made. Chapter 6 presents the proportions of women with poor pregnancy outcome and good pregnancy outcome who had diabetes complications.

Table 5.1

Characteristics of women (all figures are % unless otherwise stated)

Socio-demographic characteristics	Women in the enquiry n (%) (N=442)	Women in the CEMACH descriptive study [1] n (%) (N=3808)
Type of diabetes		
Type 1	324 (73)	2767 (73)
Type 2	118 (27)	1041 (27)
Median age at delivery (years) [IQR]	31 [25, 34]	31 [27, 35]
Ethnicity:		
White	354 (80)	3059 (80)
Black African	16 (4)	121 (3)
Black Caribbean	9 (2)	84 (2)
Black Other	0 (0)	14 (0.4)
Indian	15 (3)	110 (3)
Pakistani	24 (5)	203 (5)
Bangladeshi	8 (2)	86 (2)
Chinese	1 (0.2)	7 (0.2)
Other	13 (3)	116 (3)
Not known	2 (0.5)	8 (0.2)
Primigravidas	192 (43)	1507 (40)
Median age at onset of diabetes (years) [IQR]	19 [10, 26]	20 [11, 28]
Median duration of diabetes (years) [IQR]	9 [4, 17]	9 [4, 17]
Deprivation quintile:		
1	59 (14)	496 (14)
2	60 (15)	581 (17)
3	72 (18)	638 (18)
4	89 (22)	728 (21)
5	128 (31)	1002 (29)
Missing or resident in Wales or Northern Ireland	*34*	*363*

Table 5.2

Specific diabetes complications in women in the enquiry

Specific diabetes complication	Women in the enquiry n/N (%)
Recurrent hypoglycaemia during pregnancy	203/400 (51)
Hypoglycaemia requiring external help	63/311 (20)
Pre-existing retinopathy	73/316 (23)
New retinopathy	29/316 (9)
Nephropathy	42/359 (12)

5.3 The babies

5.3.1 Pregnancy outcomes

The outcomes of all pregnancies in the enquiry are shown in table 5.3.

Table 5.3

Outcome of pregnancies in the enquiry

	No congenital anomaly (N=315)	Congenital anomaly (N=127)	Total (N=442)
Alive at 28 days	220	66	286
Loss before 20 weeks	N/A[a]	19	19
Late fetal loss	13	26	39
Stillbirth	71	6	77
Early neonatal death	9	4	13
Late neonatal death	2	6	8

[a] Not within definition of pregnancies sampled for enquiry

Gender was known for 385 of 442 offspring. There were 192 males, 192 females and one indeterminate sex.

5.3.2 Fetal growth restriction

Thirty seven babies in the enquiry had documented antenatal evidence of fetal growth restriction or poor growth velocity (table 5.4). Seventy percent (26/37) of these babies had a poor outcome (death and/or fetal congenital anomaly) compared with 50% (222/442) of all babies in the enquiry. There was no difference in the distribution of type of diabetes or ethnicity amongst women whose babies had fetal growth restriction (table 5.4). However, 31% of the women whose babies had antenatal evidence of fetal growth restriction had nephropathy compared to 12% of women in the whole enquiry sample (p=0.002).

Table 5.4

Characteristics of women whose babies had antenatal evidence of fetal growth restriction

Maternal characteristics	Women with antenatal evidence of fetal growth restriction n (%) (N=37)	All women in the enquiry n (%) (N=442)
Type of diabetes		
Type 1	26 (70)	324 (73)
Type 2	11 (30)	118 (27)
Ethnicity		
White	31 (84)	354 (80)
Black	3 (8)	25 (6)
Asian	2 (5)	47 (11)
Chinese and Other	1 (3)	14 (3)
Median maternal age (years) [IQR]	33 [30, 34]	31 [25, 34]
Nephropathy	10/32 (31)	42/359 (12)

5.3.3 Macrosomia

One hundred and twenty nine babies had documented antenatal evidence of macrosomia (the guidance given to panels was evidence of fetal size greater than the 90th centile for gestational age). Forty one percent (53/129) of these babies had a poor outcome; this was similar to the proportion (50%, 222/442) of all babies in the enquiry having a poor outcome. There was a slightly greater proportion of type 1 diabetes and White ethnicity in women whose babies had antenatal evidence of macrosomia compared to all women in the enquiry sample, but this did not reach significance (p=0.13 and p=0.08 respectively) (table 5.5).

Table 5.5

Characteristics of women whose babies had antenatal evidence of macrosomia

Maternal characteristics	Women with antenatal evidence of fetal macrosomia n (%)[a] (N=129)	All women in the enquiry n (%) (N=442)
Type of diabetes		
Type 1	103 (80)	324 (73)
Type 2	26 (20)	118 (27)
Ethnicity		
White	112 (88)	354 (80)
Black	7 (5)	25 (6)
Asian	6 (5)	47 (10)
Chinese and Other	3 (2)	14 (3.2)
Maternal age (years) [IQR]	31 [26, 34]	31 [25, 34]
Nephropathy	10/102 (10)	42/359 (12)

[a] Percentages are the proportion of women in a category out of the total number of women with a valid response, i.e. excluding 'not applicable' and 'missing'.

5.3.4 Fetal congenital anomalies

A total of 127 offspring of women in the enquiry had a confirmed major congenital anomaly, using the European Surveillance of Congenital Anomalies (EUROCAT) classification system.[2] Over half of these babies survived beyond the neonatal period (table 5.3). Two thirds of the anomalies were detected antenatally. More details about fetal congenital anomalies in the CEMACH programme can be found elsewhere.[1,3]

5.3.5 Deaths

A total of 137 babies in the enquiry died from 20 weeks gestation up to 28 days after delivery. Forty two (31%) of these babies had a confirmed major congenital anomaly (table 5.3).

The cause of death for stillbirths and neonatal deaths (babies who died from 24 weeks of gestation up to 28 days after delivery) was categorised according to the Extended Wigglesworth classification[4] using information within the medical records, including postmortem where available. The distribution of causes of death by major category was compared to the general maternity population (table 5.6). There was a greater proportion of unexplained antepartum stillbirths amongst babies of women with diabetes than in the general maternity population. There were a greater proportion of deaths due to immaturity in the general maternity population, despite the fact that the preterm delivery rate for women with diabetes was five times higher than in the general population.[1] Further work needs to be done to investigate the possible reasons for this difference.

Table 5.6
Cause of death of stillbirths and neonatal deaths (Extended Wigglesworth classification)

Extended Wigglesworth classification*	Stillbirths and neonatal deaths in enquiry n (%) (N=98)	Stillbirths and neonatal deaths in general maternity population (2002)5 n (%) (N=5756)	P-value
Congenital defect / malformation (lethal or severe)	18 (18)	1087 (19)	0.68
Unexplained antepartum fetal death	58 (59)	2516 (44)	0.002
Death from intrapartum causes	10 (10)	429 (8)	0.30
Immaturity	4 (4)	1027 (18)	<0.001
Infection	1 (1)	252 (4)	0.10
Classification not possible from information in medical records	*7*	*36*	

* Extended Wigglesworth classification categories that were not assigned to any stillbirth or neonatal death in the enquiry, are not included in the table.

5.3.6 Postmortem examination

A postmortem examination was documented to have been offered for 89% (122/137) of babies who died. Postmortem examination was declined by parents in 39% (48/122) of cases. In ten further cases there was no information available to panels as to why the postmortem examination was not carried out despite being offered. In one case only external examination was performed, and for one case it was documented in the medical records that postmortem examination was not needed. Overall, 45% (62/137) of babies who died were documented to have had a postmortem examination, which is slightly higher than the national average of 40% in 2002-03.[5]

Postmortem examination findings were available to the panel for 57 out of 62 babies and are reported in table 5.7. The reported incidence of islet cell hyperplasia and eosinophilic infiltrates in the pancreas was lower in this group of babies than in previous reports.[6] It is difficult to be certain of the reasons for this difference, but possibilities include under-reporting due to advanced autolysis, a particular problem in the pancreas.

Table 5.7	
Postmortem examination findings in babies who died after 20 weeks gestation having a postmortem	
Specific findings reported	**n (%) (N=57)* †**
Islet cell hyperplasia	6 (11)
Eosinophilic pancreatitis	1 (2)
Cardiomegaly	10 (18)
Vascular thrombosis	0 (0)
No abnormality reported on postmortem	41 (72)

* 5 postmortem examination reports were not available.

† There may have been more than one finding reported for any baby undergoing postmortem examination.

5.4 Conclusions

Women in the enquiry were similar to women in the descriptive study with respect to socio-demographic characteristics. Due to the sampling methodology for the enquiry (see Chapter 4), half of the women in the enquiry had a poor pregnancy outcome.

Twelve percent of women in the enquiry had nephropathy and 32% had retinopathy (pre-existing or diagnosed for the first time in pregnancy). About half of women in the enquiry had recurrent hypoglycaemia during pregnancy and a fifth had at least one severe hypoglycaemic episode requiring external help.

Babies with antenatal evidence of fetal growth restriction had a higher proportion of mothers with nephropathy compared to all babies in the enquiry, and 70% had a poor outcome. Forty one per cent of babies with antenatal evidence of macrosomia had a poor outcome, which was similar to the 50% of babies in the whole enquiry sample with a poor outcome.

Sixteen percent of babies who died from 24 weeks of gestation up to 28 days after delivery had a cause of death classified as 'severe or lethal congenital anomaly'. Women in the enquiry had a higher proportion of unexplained antepartum fetal death and a lower proportion of deaths due to immaturity than the general maternity population. Nearly half of all babies who died had a postmortem examination.

References

1. *Confidential Enquiry into Maternal and Child Health. Pregnancy in women with type 1 and type 2 diabetes in 2002-03, England, Wales and Northern Ireland.* CEMACH: London; 2005.
2. *EUROCAT Report 8: Surveillance of Congenital Anomalies in Europe 1980-1999.* European Registration of Congenital Anomalies. University of Ulster: Belfast; 2002.
3. Macintosh MCM, Fleming KM, Bailey JA, Doyle P, Modder J, Acolet D, et al. *Perinatal mortality and congenital anomalies in babies of women with type 1 or type 2 diabetes in England, Wales and Northern Ireland: population based study.* BMJ 2006; 333:177.
4. *Confidential Enquiry into Stillbirths and Deaths in Infancy. 4th Annual Report 1 January – 31 December 1995.* Maternal and Child Health Research Consortium: London; 1997.
5. *Confidential Enquiry into Maternal and Child Health. Stillbirth, Neonatal and Post-neonatal Mortality 2000 – 2003, England, Wales and Northern Ireland.* CEMACH: London; 2005.
6. Jaffe R. In Wigglesworth JS, Singer DB eds. *The pancreas. Textbook of Fetal and Perinatal Pathology.* Blackwell: Massacussetts: 900-932.

6. Factors associated with poor pregnancy outcome in women with type 1 and type 2 diabetes

6.1 Introduction

Women with type 1 and type 2 diabetes continue to have an increased risk of adverse pregnancy outcomes, including miscarriage, fetal congenital anomaly and perinatal death.[1-4] A case-control approach was utilised within the enquiry module to examine the association of demographic and clinical characteristics, social and lifestyle factors and clinical care with poor pregnancy outcome.

6.2 Methodology

Poor pregnancy outcome was defined as a singleton baby with a major congenital anomaly who delivered at any gestation and/or a baby who died from 20 weeks gestation up to 28 days after delivery.

There were 222 cases that met the definition of poor pregnancy outcome. These comprised:

- Sixty one singleton babies with a major congenital anomaly who died at any gestation during pregnancy and up to 28 days after delivery. This included terminations of pregnancy for fetal congenital anomaly.
- Ninety five singleton babies without a major congenital anomaly who died from 20 weeks gestation up to 28 days after delivery.
- Sixty six babies with a major congenital anomaly who survived to 28 days after delivery.

There were 220 controls (singleton babies without a major congenital anomaly who survived to day 28 after delivery).

Odds ratios and associated 95% confidence intervals were calculated to examine each factor identified by panels and its association with adverse outcomes. Odds ratios are also displayed adjusting for maternal age and deprivation, where appropriate, to allow for the potential confounding by these factors.

6.2.1 Additional analyses

In addition to the primary analysis (section 6.2), associations of different factors with outcome were also analysed using three separate case definitions:

- All major fetal congenital anomalies
- All deaths from 20 weeks gestation up to 28 days after delivery
- Deaths from 20 weeks gestation up to 28 days after delivery, excluding major fetal congenital anomalies.

The results of these analyses can be found in Appendices C, D and E. In most cases the direction of association was the same regardless of the case definition used. Any notable differences are highlighted throughout the text.

6.3 Results

Associations of factors with poor pregnancy outcome are presented below. Each group of factors is discussed in more detail in the relevant chapter in this report.

6.3.1 Socio-demographic characteristics

Associations with poor pregnancy outcome were investigated for specific social and demographic characteristics, including age, ethnicity, social deprivation, and gravidity (table 6.1).

Table 6.1				
Association of demographic characteristics in women with type 1 and type 2 diabetes with poor pregnancy outcome				
Demographic characteristic	Cases n/N (%)	Controls n/N (%)	Crude OR [95% CI]	Adjusted OR [95% CI]
Age	-	-	1.0 [1.0, 1.0]	1.0 [1.0, 1.0][b]
Black, Asian or Other Ethnic Minority group	47/222 (21)	41/220 (19)	1.2 [0.7, 1.9]	0.9 [0.5, 1.5][a]
Primigravidity	100/222 (45)	92/220 (42)	1.1 [0.8, 1.7]	1.3 [0.9, 2.0][a]
Maternal social deprivation[d]	-	-	1.2 [1.1, 1.4]	1.2 [1.1, 1.4][c]

[a] adjusted for maternal age and deprivation.

[b] adjusted for maternal deprivation.

[c] adjusted for maternal age. Odds ratio is for one year increase in maternal age.

[d] Quintile of social deprivation derived from postcode of residence. Odds ratio is for unit increase in deprivation quintile.

Maternal deprivation was associated with poor pregnancy outcome for women with type 1 and type 2 diabetes. This was similar to the general maternity population nationally, with over one third of all stillbirths and neonatal deaths in 2004 being born to mothers resident in the most deprived quintile.[5]

However, ethnicity was not associated with poor pregnancy outcome for women in the enquiry sample, which is different to previous findings for the general maternity population.[5,6] CEMACH is committed to further investigating the contribution of ethnicity and deprivation to specific pregnancy outcomes for women with type 1 and type 2 diabetes.

6.3.2 Clinical characteristics

The clinical characteristics examined included characteristics of the women such as Body Mass Index (BMI); known complications of diabetes before pregnancy; retinopathy, nephropathy and hypoglycaemia during pregnancy; and evidence of fetal growth restriction or macrosomia during pregnancy. The results are shown in table 6.2. Women with pre-existing diabetes complications were more likely to have a poor pregnancy outcome. However, nephropathy and recurrent or severe hypoglycaemia in pregnancy were not shown to be associated with poor pregnancy outcome. Antenatal evidence of fetal growth restriction was associated with poor pregnancy outcome but antenatal evidence of fetal macrosomia was not.

Table 6.2

Association of clinical characteristics of women with type 1 and type 2 diabetes and their babies, with poor pregnancy outcome

Clinical characteristics	Cases n/N (%)	Controls n/N (%)	Crude OR [95% CI]	Adjusted OR[a] [95% CI]
Body Mass Index (BMI) ≥30	40/136 (29)	33/137 (24)	1.3 [0.8, 2.3]	1.1 [0.6, 1.9]
Pre-existing diabetes complications	37/182 (20)	16/197 (8)	2.9 [1.5, 5.5]	2.6 [1.3, 4.9]
Retinopathy in pregnancy	55/149 (37)	50/167 (30)	1.4 [0.9, 2.2]	1.4 [0.9, 2.4]
Diabetic nephropathy in pregnancy	28/174 (16)	14/185 (8)	2.3 [1.2, 4.7]	2.0 [1.0, 4.2]
Recurrent episodes of hypoglycaemia during pregnancy	98/195 (50)	105/205 (51)	1.0 [0.7, 1.4]	1.1 [0.7, 1.7]
Severe hypogylacemia during pregnancy (one or more episode of hypoglycaemia requiring external help)	31/144 (22)	32/167 (19)	1.2 [0.7, 2.0]	1.3 [0.7, 2.3]
Antenatal evidence of fetal growth restriction	26/186 (14)	11/218 (5)	3.1 [1.5, 6.4]	2.9 [1.4, 6.3]
Antenatal evidence of macrosomia (fetal size >90th centile)	53/179 (30)	76/216 (35)	0.8 [0.5, 1.2]	0.8 [0.5, 1.3]

[a] adjusted for maternal age and deprivation.

6.3.3 Social and lifestyle factors

In the enquiry, a number of social and lifestyle factors were significantly associated with poor pregnancy outcome (table 6.3), and these are further discussed in Chapter 7. There appears to be an urgent need for further research into the socio-cultural factors affecting women's behaviour; education programmes for women and health professionals; and consideration of how best to develop diabetes maternity services.

Table 6.3

Association of social and lifestyle factors in women with type 1 and type 2 diabetes with poor pregnancy outcome

Social and lifestyle factor	Cases n/N (%)	Controls n/N (%)	Crude OR [95% CI]	Adjusted OR[a] [95% CI]
Unplanned pregnancy	72/141 (51)	55/144 (38)	1.7 [1.1, 2.7]	1.8 [1.0, 2.9]
No contraceptive use in the 12 months before pregnancy	71/108 (66)	54/121 (45)	2.4 [1.4, 4.1]	2.3 [1.3, 4.0]
No folic acid commenced prior to pregnancy	83/120 (69)	66/131 (50)	2.2 [1.3, 3.8]	2.2 [1.3, 3.9]
Smoking	63/183 (34)	44/182 (24)	1.7 [1.0, 2.6]	1.9 [1.2, 3.2]
Assessment of suboptimal approach of the woman to managing her diabetes before pregnancy	137/160 (83)	88/154 (57)	4.5 [2.5, 7.9]	4.9 [2.7, 8.8]
Assessment of suboptimal approach of the woman to managing her diabetes during pregnancy	118/197 (60)	56/207 (27)	4.0 [2.6, 6.3]	3.9 [2.5, 6.1]

[a] adjusted for maternal age and deprivation.

6.3.4 Glycaemic control

A test of glycaemic control before pregnancy, local glycaemic control targets, and panel assessments of glycaemic control before and during pregnancy, were examined in relation to poor pregnancy outcome (table 6.4). A lack of local glycaemic control targets, and suboptimal glycaemic control before and during pregnancy were associated with poor pregnancy outcome. These issues are discussed further in Chapters 7 and 8.

Table 6.4

Association of factors related to glycaemic control before and during pregnancy in women with type 1 and type 2 diabetes, with poor pregnancy outcome

Factor related to glycaemic control	Cases n/N (%)	Controls n/N (%)	Crude OR [95% CI]	Adjusted OR[a] [95% CI]
No test of glycaemic control in the 12 months prior to pregnancy	36/139 (26)	24/139 (17)	1.7 [0.9, 3.0]	1.5 [0.8, 2.8]
No local targets set for glycaemic control	44/90 (49)	28/86 (33)	2.0 [1.1, 3.7]	2.0 [1.0, 3.8]
Assessment of suboptimal preconception glycaemic control	165/187 (88)	115/167 (69)	3.4 [1.9, 6.0]	3.9 [2.2, 7.0]
Assessment of suboptimal 1st trimester glycaemic control	171/204 (84)	118/192 (61)	3.3 [2.0, 5.3]	3.4 [2.1, 5.7]
Assessment of suboptimal glycaemic control after 1st trimester	146/205 (71)	76/209 (37)	4.3 [2.8, 6.7]	5.2 [3.3, 8.2]
Assessment of suboptimal glycaemic control during labour and delivery	80/162 (49)	96/202 (48)	0.9 [0.6, 1.4]	1.0 [0.7, 1.6]
No intravenous insulin and dextrose during labour and/or delivery	48/208 (23)	31/217 (14)	1.8 [1.1, 3.0]	1.8 [1.1, 3.0]

[a] adjusted for maternal age and deprivation.

6.3.5 Preconception care in the 12 months prior to pregnancy

Specific preconception care factors, based on the medical records held by adult diabetes services or general practitioners, were investigated for association with poor pregnancy outcome. The results are shown in table 6.5 and are discussed further in chapter 8. These findings were dependent on documentation in the medical records, and poor documentation by health professionals of the care and advice given to women may have influenced the apparent association with poor pregnancy outcome.

Table 6.5

Association of specific preconception care factors in women with type 1 and type 2 diabetes with poor pregnancy outcome

Preconception care factor	Cases n/N (%)	Controls n/N (%)	Crude OR [95% CI]	Adjusted OR[a] [95% CI]
No contraceptive advice provided before pregnancy	28/85 (33)	19/83 (23)	1.7 [0.8, 3.3]	1.7 [0.8, 3.5]
No discussion of the following specific diabetes issues:				
Alcohol intake	31/70 (44)	19/66 (29)	2.0 [1.0, 4.1]	2.5 [1.1, 5.4]
Diet	20/103 (19)	12/100 (12)	1.8 [0.8, 3.9]	1.8 [0.8, 4.1]
Poor glycaemic control	18/118 (15)	14/117 (12)	1.3 [0.6, 2.8]	1.2 [0.5, 2.5]
Retinopathy	25/83 (30)	25/96 (26)	1.2 [0.6, 2.4]	1.1 [0.6, 2.3]
Nephropathy	28/74 (38)	29/76 (38)	1.0 [0.5, 1.9]	0.8 [0.4, 1.7]
Hypertension	27/71 (38)	23/75 (31)	1.4 [0.7, 2.8]	1.1 [0.5, 2.3]
No discussion of the following pregnancy issues:				
Increased diabetes surveillance	13/123 (11)	7/124 (6)	2.0 [0.8, 5.2]	1.7 [0.6, 4.5]
Increased pregnancy surveillance	13/117 (11)	8/124 (6)	1.8 [0.7, 4.6]	1.5 [0.6, 4.0]
Increased risk of induction	21/83 (25)	14/110 (13)	2.3 [1.1, 5.0]	2.2 [1.0, 4.9]
Possible caesarean section	20/95 (21)	11/110 (10)	2.4 [1.1, 5.4]	2.4 [1.0, 5.8]
Fetal risks in diabetic pregnancy	17/98 (17)	7/114 (6)	3.2 [1.3, 8.2]	2.9 [1.1, 8.2]
No dietetic review	46/129 (36)	42/135 (61)	1.2 [0.7, 2.1]	1.2 [0.7, 2.1]
No assessment of the following diabetes complications in the 12 months prior to pregnancy:				
Baseline retinal examination	36/141 (26)	18/137 (13)	2.3 [1.2, 4.3]	2.3 [1.2, 4.5]
Baseline test of renal function	26/130 (20)	15/133 (11)	2.0 [1.0, 3.9]	2.0 [0.9, 4.3]
Assessment of albuminuria	41/116 (35)	30/109 (28)	1.4 [0.8, 2.6]	1.5 [0.8, 2.8]
Assessment of suboptimal preconception care (excluding glycaemic control)	116/133 (87)	80/134 (60)	4.6 [2.4, 8.8]	5.2 [2.7, 10.1]

[a] adjusted for maternal age and deprivation.

6.3.6 Diabetes care (excluding glycaemic control)

Diabetes care in the enquiry referred to monitoring for diabetes complications, including retinal assessments and tests of renal function. Findings are shown in table 6.6 and are discussed further in Chapter 9.

Table 6.6

Association of diabetes care factors (excluding glycaemic control) in women with type 1 and type 2 diabetes, with poor pregnancy outcome

Diabetes care factor	Cases n/N (%)	Controls n/N (%)	Crude OR [95% CI]	Adjusted OR[a] [95% CI]
No retinal assessment during first trimester or at booking if later	70/194 (36)	49/183 (27)	1.5 [1.0, 2.4]	1.4 [0.9, 2.2]
No referral to ophthalmologist (if retinopathy present)	10/45 (22)	21/44 (48)	0.3 [0.1, 0.8]	0.2 [0.1, 0.7]
No monitoring for nephropathy	46/209 (22)	26/206 (13)	2.0 [1.2, 3.3]	1.9 [1.1, 3.3]
No test of renal function (if nephropathy present)	12/26 (46)	5/14 (36)	1.5 [0.4, 6.0]	1.9 [0.3, 6.0]
Assessment of suboptimal diabetes care during pregnancy	146/204 (72)	118/204 (58)	1.8 [1.2, 2.8]	1.7 [1.1, 2.6]

[a] adjusted for maternal age and deprivation.

6.3.7 Maternity care

The association of maternity care factors with poor pregnancy outcome are shown in table 6.7. It is of concern that suboptimal maternity care during pregnancy and suboptimal antenatal fetal surveillance of big babies were associated with poor pregnancy outcome. This, together with issues relating to discussion of mode and timing of delivery, are discussed further in Chapter 9.

Table 6.7

Association of maternity care factors in women with type 1 and type 2 diabetes with poor pregnancy outcome

Maternity care factor	Cases n/N (%)	Controls n/N (%)	Crude OR [95% CI]	Adjusted OR [95% CI]
Assessment of suboptimal fetal monitoring (with antenatal evidence of growth restricted baby)	6/24 (25)	1/11 (9)	3.3 [0.3, 34.1]	2.3 [0.2, 26.3]
Assessment of suboptimal fetal monitoring (with antenatal evidence of fetal size > 90th centile)	35/52 (67)	27/73 (37)	3.5 [1.7, 7.4]	5.3 [2.4, 12.0]
No discussion of mode and timing of delivery	15/178 (8)	4/202 (2)	4.6 [1.5, 14.2]	4.0 [1.2, 12.7]
No administration of antenatal corticosteroids [b]	14/41 (34)	12/33 (36)	0.9 [0.4, 2.4]	0.9 [0.3, 2.5]
Assessment of suboptimal maternity care during the antenatal period	125/215 (58)	95/215 (44)	1.8 [1.2, 2.6]	1.9 [1.2, 2.8]
Assessment of suboptimal maternity care during labour and delivery	78/199 (39)	72/213 (34)	1.3 [0.8, 1.9]	1.3 [0.8, 1.9]

[a] adjusted for maternal age and deprivation.

[b] Analysis restricted to babies delivering from 24+0 to 35+6 weeks gestation and excluding antepartum stillbirths.

6.3.8 Postnatal care

Although postnatal care factors could not have been causative to poor pregnancy outcome, women who had a poor pregnancy outcome were more likely to have suboptimal postnatal diabetes care and no contraceptive advice before discharge from hospital (table 6.8). This is discussed further in Chapter 9.

Table 6.8

Association of postnatal care factors with poor pregnancy outcome in women with type 1 and type 2 diabetes

Postnatal care factor	Cases n/N (%)	Controls n/N (%)	Crude OR [95% CI]	Adjusted OR[a] [95% CI]
No postnatal contraceptive advice	63/143 (44)	26/163 (16)	4.2 [2.4, 7.3]	4.2 [2.4, 7.4]
No written plan for post-delivery diabetes management	31/184 (17)	25/188 (13)	1.3 [0.8, 2.3]	1.4 [0.8, 2.6]
Assessment of suboptimal postnatal diabetes care	133/203 (66)	106/211 (50)	1.9 [1.3, 2.8]	1.8 [1.2, 2.7]

[a] adjusted for maternal age and deprivation.

6.4 Conclusions

The case-control analysis has noted a number of associations between demographic, social and lifestyle factors and clinical care with poor pregnancy outcome, and these are discussed further in the relevant chapters in this report. It should be noted that these factors are based on documentation in the medical records and on panels' assessment of behaviour or care, which introduce potential problems, firstly with the high proportion of missing results for some data items, and secondly with potential bias due to lack of blinding of the panel assessors. There may also be confounding factors and although attempts have been made to adjust for some of these in the analysis, there may still be other factors that have not been taken into account. Overall, however, the findings support the argument that preparation for pregnancy, glycaemic control, and the standard of preconception and pregnancy care need to be improved if better pregnancy outcomes are to be achieved for women with diabetes.

References

1. Macintosh M, Fleming K, Bailey J, Doyle P, Modder J, Acolet D, et al. *Perinatal mortality and congenital anomalies in babies of women with type 1 or type 2 diabetes in England, Wales and Northern Ireland: population based study.* BMJ, Jul 22 2006 333 (7560):177.
2. Evers I, de Valk H, Visser G. *Risk of complications of pregnancy in women with type 1 diabetes: nationwide prospective study in the Netherlands.* BMJ, Apr 17 2004 328(7445):915.
3. Verheijen E, Critchley J, Whitelaw D, Tuffnell D. *Outcomes of pregnancies in women with pre-existing type 1 or type 2 diabetes, in an ethnically mixed population.* BJOG, Nov 2005 112(11):1500-3.
4. Jensen D, Damm P, Moelsted-Pedersen L, Ovesen P, Westergaard J, Moeller M, et al. *Outcomes in type 1 diabetic pregnancies: a nationwide, population-based study.* Diabetes Care, Dec 2004 27(12):2819-23.
5. *Confidential Enquiry into Maternal and Child Health. Perinatal Mortality Surveillance, 2004: England, Wales and Northern Ireland.* CEMACH: London; 2006.
6. Collingwood Bakeo A. *Investigating variations in infant mortality in England and Wales by mother's country of birth, 1983 – 2001.* Paediatric and Perinatal Epidemiology, Mar 2006 20(2):127-39.

7. Social and lifestyle issues

Learning points

- Women with diabetes do not appear to be adequately prepared for pregnancy.
- Two thirds of women with diabetes had suboptimal glycaemic control before and during the first trimester of pregnancy.
- Suboptimal glycaemic control before and during pregnancy, and a suboptimal approach of the woman to managing her diabetes, were associated with poor pregnancy outcome.
- The main underlying issues for women with diabetes were:
  - non-attendance at planned appointments
  - non-adherence to medical advice about diabetes management
  - unplanned pregnancy
  - social factors including language difficulties and domestic circumstances.

7.1 Introduction

The prevalence of diabetes in the UK is increasing, with an increasing number of young people being diagnosed.[1-3] There are an estimated 131 000 women diagnosed with diabetes of childbearing age in England *(Diabetes UK, personal communication)* . The CEMACH report on 3808 pregnancies to women with type 1 and type 2 diabetes has shown that women in England, Wales and Northern Ireland are poorly prepared for pregnancy.[4]

This chapter examines some of the underlying issues that were identified during panel reviews of 442 singleton pregnancies to women with diabetes in England, Wales and Northern Ireland.

7.2 Preparation for pregnancy

Development of the fetal organs occurs during the first three months of pregnancy, and there is evidence that good glycaemic control in the preconception period and during the first trimester of pregnancy decreases the risk of fetal congenital anomaly and miscarriage.[5-7] Women with diabetes of childbearing age need to use an effective and reliable method of contraception to avoid unplanned pregnancy, and it is recommended that women planning a pregnancy should continue contraception until good glycaemic control has been achieved.[8] In addition, it has been shown that high dose (5mg) folic acid commenced before pregnancy decreases the risk of fetal neural tube defects in high risk populations[9] and this is recommended for women with diabetes.[1,10] Smoking increases the risk of diabetes vascular complications and placental insufficiency, and women should be advised and encouraged to stop smoking.

7.2.1 Enquiry findings

Less than half (41%, 158/384) of women in the enquiry (35% of 197 cases[a] and 48% of 187 controls[b]) were documented to have planned their current pregnancy, compared to a planned pregnancy rate of 58% in 2001-02 in the general maternity population.[11] Twenty seven percent (107/32) of women (19% of 196 cases and 36% of 196 controls) were documented to have been using any form of contraception in the 12 months before conception. Twenty seven percent of 380 women were documented to have commenced folic acid before pregnancy (19% of 193 cases and 35% of 187 controls). This is comparable to the general maternity population in the UK, where the uptake of folic acid has been shown to range from less than 10% to 50% in different studies.[12] Only 33 women were documented to be on high dose (5mg daily) folic acid.

Women who did not have a record of any form of contraceptive use in the 12 months before pregnancy were more likely to have a poor pregnancy outcome (OR 2.3, 95% CI 1.3 - 4.0 adjusted for maternal age and deprivation, see Chapter 6). In the additional case-control analysis (see Appendices C, D and E) the specific association was with fetal or neonatal death from 20 weeks gestation and not with fetal congenital anomaly. This suggests that these women were not aware of the importance of using contraception until optimal glycaemic control had been achieved prior to conception, and may have been unaware of the importance of good pregnancy preparation in order to reduce the risks of adverse pregnancy outcomes.

Twenty eight percent (107/386) of women with diabetes were documented as smoking before pregnancy (32% of 197 cases and 23% of 189 controls). This compares to a rate of 35% in the general maternity population.[11]

7.3 Panel assessment of glycaemic control

Optimal glycaemic control before and during pregnancy is one of the main principles of management for women with pre-existing diabetes, as this decreases the risk of adverse pregnancy outcomes. [5-7] This can be challenging for women who already have to cope with the ongoing demands of their diabetes, and health professionals and women need to work in partnership to achieve good control.

The guidance given to enquiry panels was that optimal glycaemic control before and during pregnancy referred to an HbA1c of less than 7%. However, it was emphasised that panel assessors may have additional information available to them at enquiry, and in this case should base their assessment on all the available information.

Enquiry panels assessed that 64% of 440 women (74% of 222 cases and 53% of 218 of controls) had suboptimal glycaemic control before pregnancy and 66% of 439 women (77% of 222 cases and 54% of 217 controls) had suboptimal control during the first trimester of pregnancy. After the first trimester and up to labour and delivery, this decreased to 51% of 443 women (68% of 215 cases and 35% of 218 controls) of women with continuing pregnancies. Suboptimal glycaemic control before and during pregnancy was associated with poor pregnancy outcome (OR 3.9, 95% CI 2.2 - 7.0 pre-pregnancy; OR 3.4, 95% CI 2.1 - 5.7 in first trimester; OR 5.2 , 95% CI 3.3 - 8.2 after first trimester (all OR adjusted for maternal age and deprivation, see Chapter 6).

[a] In this chapter, a case refers to a woman who had a poor pregnancy outcome, defined as a singleton baby with a major congenital anomaly who delivered at any gestation and/or a baby who died from 20 weeks gestation up to 28 days after delivery.

[b] In this chapter, a control refers to a woman who had a good pregnancy outcome, defined as a singleton baby without a congenital anomaly who survived to day 28 after delivery.

7.3.1 Panel comments on suboptimal preconception glycaemic control

Enquiry panels made a total of 334 comments for 280 women with suboptimal preconception glycaemic control. The majority of these comments related to social and lifestyle issues (table 7.1). Twenty percent of women with suboptimal glycaemic control did not attend planned appointments, Ten percent had an unplanned pregnancy and 19% did not follow advice about the management of their diabetes. Eleven percent of women were socially vulnerable (mainly language difficulties and domestic circumstances) or had erratic or busy lifestyles.

Table 7.1

Panel comments on suboptimal preconception glycaemic control (table contains information following categorisation of free text)

	Women with suboptimal preconception glycaemic control			
	Good pregnancy outcome (N=115)		Poor pregnancy outcome (N=165)	
	No. of comments	% of women	No. of comments	% of women
Total comments[a]	*68*		*119*	
Medical, social and lifestyle factors[b]	32	-	48	-
Unplanned pregnancy	12	10	16	10
Social vulnerability or lifestyle problems	9	8	22	13
Medical factors	11	10	9	5
Poor education / understanding of diabetes	0	-	1	1
Woman did not attend appointments	14	12	41	25
Non adherence to diet, HBGM[c] **or insulin**	22	19	30	18

[a] There were 81 additional comments where the issues were not described by panels; 18 comments where there was a lack of preconception care with the reason being unclear to panels; and 48 comments about clinical care. These comments are not included in the table.

[b] A single woman could have more than one comment in the medical, social and lifestyle category, therefore % of women calculated only for individual factors.

[c] Home blood glucose monitoring.

7.3.2 Panel comments on suboptimal glycaemic control during pregnancy

Panels made a total of 154 comments about social and lifestyle issues in the first trimester and 94 comments about social and lifestyle issues in the second trimester . The main issues were non-adherence to medical advice and failure to attend planned appointments. 'Medical, lifestyle or social factors' included concerns about erratic lifestyles and social problems (table 7.2).

Table 7.2

Panel comments on social and lifestyle issues underlying suboptimal glycaemic control during pregnancy in women with pre-existing diabetes (table contains information following categorisation of free text)

	Women assessed to have suboptimal glycaemic control in the 1st trimester				Women assessed to have suboptimal glycaemic control after the 1st trimester			
	Good pregnancy outcome (N=118)		Poor pregnancy outcome (N=171)		Good pregnancy outcome (N=76)		Poor pregnancy outcome (N=146)	
	No. of comments	% of women	No. of comments	% of women	No. of comments	% of women	No. of comments	% of women
Total comments*	57	-	97	-	27	-	67	-
Non adherence to medical advice	19	16	36	21	11	14	20	10
Medical, lifestyle or social factors	8	7	9	5	4	5	11	8
Duration and severity of diabetes	6	5	8	5	4	5	10	7
Woman did not attend planned appointments	10	8	21	12	5	7	14	10
Actively chose not to follow medical advice	1	1	3	2	3	4	6	4
Late booker	6	5	14	8	0	0	0	0
Unplanned pregnancy	7	6	6	4	0	0	0	0

* There were 178 comments made about clinical care issues; these comments are not included in this table but are included in table 9.1 (Chapter 9).

7.4 Women's approach to managing their diabetes

Women with diabetes may have an increased burden on their work and personal lives both before and during pregnancy, due to the additional issues which arise at this time. This can sometimes lead to a suboptimal approach to managing their diabetes.

7.4.1 Panel assessment of women's approach to managing their diabetes

Enquiry panels assessed that 51% of 434 women had a suboptimal approach to managing their diabetes before pregnancy (62% of 216 cases and 40% of 218 controls) and 40% of 434 women had a suboptimal approach to managing their diabetes during pregnancy (55% of 216 cases and 26% of 218 controls). A suboptimal approach of the woman to managing her diabetes either before or during pregnancy was associated with poor pregnancy outcome (OR 4.9, 95% CI 2.7 - 8.8 and OR 3.9 , 95% CI 2.5 - 6.1 respectively, adjusted for maternal age and deprivation, see Chapter 6).

7.4.2 Panel comments on suboptimal approach of the woman to managing her diabetes

Panels made 283 comments for 222 women before pregnancy and 199 comments for 174 women during pregnancy (table 7.3). The main issues were non-adherence to medical advice, non-attendance at planned appointments, and social factors including unplanned pregnancy, poor motivation and poor understanding of diabetes.

Table 7.3 Panel comments on suboptimal approach of the woman to managing her diabetes (table contains information following categorisation of free text)	Women assessed to have suboptimal approach to diabetes management before pregnancy				Women assessed to have suboptimal approach to diabetes management during pregnancy			
	Good pregnancy outcome (N=88)		Poor pregnancy outcome (N=134)		Good pregnancy outcome (N=56)		Poor pregnancy outcome (N=118)	
	No. of comments	% of women	No. of comments	% of women	No. of comments	% of women	No. of comments	% of women
*Total comments**	*110*		*167*		*65*		*106*	
Medical, lifestyle, social factors[†]	**42**	-	**65**	-	**16**	-	**38**	-
Unplanned pregnancy or no contraception	14	16	22	16	1	2	2	2
Poorly motivated	8	9	8	6	4	7	2	2
Poor education or understanding of diabetes	3	3	6	4	3	5	4	3
Other social or lifestyle factors	15	17	29	22	4	7	16	14
Medical factors	2	2	0	-	4	7	14	12
Non-adherence to medical advice	32	36	45	34	27	48	38	32
Woman did not attend appointments	25	28	46	34	13	23	18	15
Woman actively chose not to follow medical advice	8	9	7	5	7	13	9	8
Duration or severity of diabetes	3	3	4	3	2	4	3	3

* There were 6 comments on clinical care before pregnancy and 28 comments on clinical care during pregnancy; these comments are not included in the table.

† A single woman could have more than one comment in the medical, social and lifestyle category, therefore % of women calculated only for individual factors.

7.5 Conclusions

One of the key findings of the previous CEMACH report[4] was that women with diabetes in England, Wales and Northern Ireland are poorly prepared for pregnancy, and many enter pregnancy with poor glycaemic control. Further exploration of the underlying issues for the 442 women in the enquiry has confirmed that two thirds of women had suboptimal glycaemic control before and in early pregnancy, as assessed by enquiry panels. It is of concern that the main underlying factors appeared to be social issues and women's approach to managing their diabetes.

Suboptimal glycaemic control and a suboptimal approach by women to diabetes management is associated with poor pregnancy outcome (see Chapter 6), and the above issues need to be considered as a matter of urgency if education programmes and preconception services are to reach those women who need support to improve their pregnancy outcomes. Further research is needed into the possible social, cultural and emotional factors affecting women's preconception behaviour and how these can be addressed. Primary and secondary care providers are likely to need to work together with local communities in order to engage with women with diabetes before they enter pregnancy.

Some quotes from the panel discussions

Social and lifestyle issues:

- 'HbA1c 8.8. Communication problems (husband acted as interpreter). Cultural problems: woman fasting during festivals. Suspected educational problems.'
- 'HbA1c 9.3 at 4 weeks. Patient not monitoring. Overseas refugee, language difficulties'.
- 'Lifestyle – hours of work - busy life.'
- 'Her obesity, social factors 'domestic turmoil'. No evidence of regular diabetes review - seems to have lost contact with professionals.'
- 'Unplanned pregnancy'.
- Non-adherence to medical advice:
- 'patient did not take dietary recommendations and did not take insulin regularly'.
- 'HbA1c pre-pregnancy range 11.5 - 7.4%, but non-compliant with diet, forgets injection, regular hypo's, lack of carbohydrates.'
- 'patient did not test her levels for optimal care (average three per week)'.

Non-attendance at planned appointments:

- 'No pre-pregnancy care. 5 appointments sent by midwife and DSN. Not checking blood sugars'.
- 'Inconsistent attendances at clinic. ? Lifestyle problems - single mother with 2 small children'.
- HBA1c 10.4 at booking, brittle diabetic disease process. Woman was poor attender. Diabetic coma three months prior to pregnancy'.

7.6 Recommendations

Clinical

1. Preconception and maternity services related to pregnancy should be easily accessible and responsive to all women with diabetes, and provide appropriate care and information.
2. There should be mechanisms in place to identify vulnerable communities and individuals, so that additional services can be provided as appropriate to women of childbearing age with diabetes, thereby ensuring optimal preconception care.
3. Providers of diabetes care should develop educational strategies that will enable all women of childbearing age with diabetes to prepare adequately for pregnancy .

Audit and research

4. Research should be carried out to:
   - identify the barriers to accessing preconception care
   - identify possible strategies to support self-care and pregnancy planning by women with diabetes.

References

1. *National Service Framework for Diabetes (England) Standards.* Department of Health: The Stationery Office: London 2001.
2. Newham A, Ryan R. *Prevalence of diagnosed diabetes mellitus in general practice in England and Wales, 1994 to 1998.* Health Statistics Quarterly 14 Summer 2002.
3. *The emergence of type 2 diabetes in childhood.* Ehtisham S. Annals of Clinical Biochemistry 41(Pt1), Jan 2004: 10-6.
4. *Confidential Enquiry into Maternal and Child Health. Pregnancy in women with type 1 and type 2 diabetes in 2002-03, England, Wales and Northern Ireland.* CEMACH: London; 2005.
5. *Pregnancy outcomes in the Diabetes Complications Trial.* The Diabetes Control and Complications Trial Research Group. Am J Obstet Gynecol; 1996 174: 1343-53.
6. Suhonen L, Hiilesmaa V, Teramo K. *Glycaemic control during early pregnancy and fetal malformations in women with type 1 diabetes mellitus..* Diabetologia 2000; 43:79-82.
7. Kitzmiller JL, Gavin LA, Gin GD et al. *Preconception care of diabetes. Glycemic control prevents congenital anomalies.* JAMA: 1991 265: 731-6.
8. *Diabetes UK Care Recommendation. Preconception care for women with diabetes.* [http://www.diabetes.org.uk/About_us/Our_Views/Care_recommendations/Preconception_care_for_women_with_diabetes/] accessed 9 December 2006.
9. Lumley J, Watson L, Watson M, Bower C. *Periconceptional supplementation with folate and/or multivitamins for preventing neural tube defects.* Cochrane Pregnancy and Childbirth Group. Cochrane Database of Systematic Reviews, 2006 3.
10. *Diabetes UK Care Recommendation. Folic acid supplementation in pregnancy. June 2005* [http://www.diabetes.org.uk/About_us/Our_Views/Care_recommendations/Folic_acid/supplementation_in_pregnancy/] accessed 9 December 2006.

11. Dex S, Heather J (eds). *Millennium Cohort Study First Survey: a user's guide to initial findings.* Centre for Longitudinal Studies: London; 2004.
12. Ray JG, Singh G, Burrows RF. *Evidence for suboptimal use of periconceptional folic acid supplements globally.* BJOG 2004;111:399-408.

Commentary

Kirsty Samuel

CEMACH lay panel assessor, Legal assessor, woman with type 1 diabetes and mother of two children.

As a lay panel assessor in the CEMACH diabetes enquiry, a woman with diabetes and a mother of two children, I feel this chapter highlights a number of important areas in explaining the unacceptably high number of adverse pregnancy outcomes for women with diabetes. However it is the reasons behind the figures that are of relevance in going forward. Why is suboptimal glycaemic control before and during pregnancy so common and why is the woman's approach to managing her diabetes less than ideal? These two questions are, in my opinion, inextricably linked. The answer lies in the lack of accessible diabetes education and pre-pregnancy counselling. Women do not realise the importance of good control, and therefore do not 'follow the advice given', as it does not seem either significant or achievable to them.

Women with diabetes of childbearing age need to be made more aware of the potential impact of poor glycaemic control on pregnancy outcomes. This information should be made available before pregnancy is seriously contemplated so that HbA1c levels can be reduced in preparation for pregnancy and unplanned pregnancies can be avoided. Women with type 2 diabetes particularly need to be targeted as many wrongly believe that their condition is less serious than type 1 diabetes and therefore will have less of an impact on pregnancy.

In conjunction with this counselling, women need to be told of the tangible benefits of good control and the greatly increased likelihood of having a healthy baby, as fear of complications and congenital anomalies also has a part to play in non-attendance at clinics.

As optimal glycaemic control is central to diabetes management in pregnancy, the means to achieve it has to be provided more effectively. The practicalities of attaining near perfect control for such a long period of time are frightening and off-putting to many women, who find good control hard enough to achieve without the additional burden of pregnancy. Realistic targets must be set, and ongoing support and reassurance provided. Women need to know that their blood sugar levels will fluctuate, and should be taught how to deal with these fluctuations in practical terms - how to adjust their insulin, when and how to test their urine for ketones, and when to seek medical help. This will require a great deal of additional support and resources but by teaching women how to manage their glycaemic control more effectively, they will feel more involved, more secure and more able to deal with the realities of pregnancy.

Non-attendance at appointments will hopefully decrease in the future with increased public knowledge and awareness of the importance of adhering to medical advice. However this, along with a fear of being 'told off' for failing to meet targets, is only one element of non-attendance at clinics. Practical problems such as long waiting times, especially for women with children, must be addressed. If more women actually saw all the relevant physicians during one clinic appointment this would reduce the time spent at the hospital, the burden of multiple appointments, and would increase women's motivation to attend further appointments.

The findings of this report all point to the need for a widespread diabetes education programme for all women with type 1 and type 2 diabetes of childbearing age and the development of an effective preconception service. While many women are far from 'perfect' in terms of knowledge, attitude and co-operation, this can only change in a significant way if the basic education and support systems are in place. Women need to have the knowledge, and the means to achieve good control, so that they can increase their chances of a positive pregnancy outcome.

8. Clinical care issues: preconception

Learning points

- In the CEMACH survey of maternity services, only 17% of maternity units in England, Wales and Northern Ireland reported providing structured multidisciplinary preconception care for women with diabetes. A quarter of women in the enquiry were reported to have had preconception care at a multidisciplinary hospital clinic.

- Two thirds of women in the enquiry had suboptimal preconception care. One of the main underlying issues was failure of health professionals to provide appropriate care such as preconception advice and higher dose folic acid. There was poor documentation of pre-pregnancy counselling.

- Suboptimal preconception care was associated with poor pregnancy outcome.

8.1 Introduction

Women with type 1 and type 2 diabetes represent a high-risk population during pregnancy. Clinicians have a responsibility to provide appropriate information, effective fetal and maternal surveillance, and timely health care interventions to achieve the best possible outcome for the woman and her baby. The Diabetes National Service Framework (NSF) emphasises the importance of an effective multidisciplinary team, both to support and empower women to plan their pregnancies, optimise glycaemic control before conception and improve the quality of antenatal care during pregnancy.[1] However, the recent CEMACH descriptive study of 3808 pregnancies to women with type 1 and type 2 diabetes found that the majority of women with pre-existing diabetes in England, Wales and Northern Ireland are poorly prepared for pregnancy.[2]

8.2 Preconception care services

The increased risk of fetal congenital anomalies (with the main contributors being neural tube and cardiac defects)[3] and perinatal death in babies of women with pre-existing diabetes[2] can be minimised by ensuring good glycaemic control before and during pregnancy[4] and by commencing high dose (5mg daily) folic acid before conception.[5]

During the CEMACH survey of maternity services (2004)[6] , only 17% of maternity units in England, Wales and Northern Ireland reported that they provided a multidisciplinary diabetes preconception service. The CEMACH descriptive study found that only 35% of women were documented in the medical notes to have had pre-pregnancy counselling, with only a tenth of these seen in a formal preconception clinic.[2] During the enquiry, general practitioners and adult diabetes services were also asked where preconception care had been provided.

8.2.1 Enquiry findings

28% of 442 women in the enquiry were reported to have had preconception care in the adult diabetes clinic and 15% with their general practitioner. 26% were reported to have had care at a hospital multidisciplinary clinic, although it was not specified as to whether this included a maternity component. For a further 4% the venue of preconception care was reported as 'other'. Information about where preconception care was provided was not available for 27% of 442 women.

8.3 Pre-pregnancy counselling

Women need to be aware of the importance of pregnancy planning, good glycaemic control, and screening for specific diabetes complications before pregnancy, and should be supported to have a healthy diet and lifestyle. They are also more likely than the general maternity population to have medical intervention during pregnancy[1,2] and this may be perceived as negative or frightening unless it is discussed at an early stage. It is therefore important to discuss pregnancy risks, planned pregnancy surveillance and any possible interventions, in the preconception period.

For each woman, the general practitioner or adult diabetes service was asked if there was documented evidence that these issues had been discussed in the 12 months before pregnancy.

8.3.1 Enquiry findings

Just over half (53%, 203/382) of women in the enquiry were documented to have had a discussion about glycaemic control before pregnancy. Forty five percent of 382 women were recorded to have had a discussion about diet and 46% of 380 women to have been reviewed by a dietitian before pregnancy. Contraception was recorded to have been discussed with only 32% of 380 women. Documentation of discussion about specific diabetes complications ranged from 24% of 381 women for nephropathy to 34% of 380 women for retinopathy. Alcohol intake was discussed with just over a fifth of women (table 8.1).

Table 8.1

Diabetes-related issues discussed with women before pregnancy

Specific issue discussed	Women with poor pregnancy outcome n/N (%)	Women with good pregnancy outcome n/N (%)	All women in the enquiry n/N (%)
Glycaemic control	100/197 (51)	103/185 (56)	203/382 (53)
Diet	83/196 (42)	88/185 (48)	171/381 (45)
Retinopathy	58/196 (30)	71/184 (39)	129/380 (34)
Contraception	37/196 (19)	67/186 (36)	121/382 (32)
Hypertension	44/196 (22)	52/184 (28)	96/380 (25)
Nephropathy	46/196 (23)	47/185 (25)	93/381 (24)
Alcohol intake	39/196 (20)	47/185 (25)	86/381 (23)

Sixty percent of 381 women (54% of 191 cases[a] and 62% of 187 controls[b]) were recorded to have had a discussion about the need for increased pregnancy surveillance. However, discussion about fetal risks was documented for just 50% of 380 women (42% of 194 cases and 58% of 186 controls). The increased chance of induction of labour was recorded as discussed with 42% of 380 women (32% of 193 cases and 51% of 107 controls), and the possibility of caesarean delivery was recorded as discussed with 46% of 381 women (39% of 194 cases and 53% of 187 controls). Women who did not have a discussion about fetal risks and the possibility of caesarean delivery were more likely to have a poor pregnancy outcome (OR 2.9, 95% CI 1.1, 8.2; and 2.4, 95% CI 1.0– 5.8 respectively, adjusted for maternal age and deprivation, see Chapter 6). Additional case-control analysis (see Appendices C, D and E) showed that the specific association was with fetal or neonatal death from 20 weeks gestation and not with fetal congenital anomaly. Women who did not receive appropriate information about the risks and strategies of management before pregnancy may have been less aware of the importance of optimal glycaemic control and the need for careful diabetes management through pregnancy.

[a] In this chapter, a case refers to a woman who had a poor pregnancy outcome, defined as a singleton baby with a major congenital anomaly who delivered at any gestation and/or a baby who died from 20 weeks gestation up to 28 days after delivery.

[b] In this chapter, a control refers to a woman who had a good pregnancy outcome, defined as a singleton baby without a congenital anomaly who survived to day 28 after delivery.

8.4 Screening for diabetes complications

Pregnancy can cause deterioration of diabetes complications such as retinopathy and renal disease, and screening for diabetes complications should be undertaken so that any necessary treatment can be provided prior to pregnancy.

8.4.1 Enquiry findings

In the year before pregnancy, only 59% of 382 women (54% of 196 cases and 64% of 186 controls) had a retinal examination, and 58% of 382 women (53% of 195 cases and 63% of 187 controls) had a renal function test (creatinine, electrolytes and urea). Women who did not have a retinal examination in the year before pregnancy were more likely to have a poor pregnancy outcome (OR 2.3, 95% CI 1.2 - 4.5, adjusted for maternal age and deprivation, see Chapter 6). In the additional case-control analysis (see Appendices C, D and E) the specific association was with fetal or neonatal death from 20 weeks gestation and not with fetal congenital anomaly. These women may have been less likely to access diabetes services before pregnancy, either for cultural and societal reasons or due to inaccessible services; and may not have been aware of the importance of pregnancy preparation and the risks of diabetic pregnancy.

8.5 Panel assessment of preconception care

The enquiry panels assessed that 73% of 267 women (87% of 133 cases and 60% of 134 controls) had suboptimal preconception care. Women having suboptimal care were more likely to go on to have a poor pregnancy outcome (OR 5.2, 95% CI 2.7 - 10.1, adjusted for maternal age and deprivation, see Chapter 6). Additional case-control analysis (see Appendices C, D and E) showed an association with fetal congenital anomaly but not with fetal or neonatal death from 20 weeks in babies without a congenital anomaly.

8.5.1 Panel comments on suboptimal preconception care

Enquiry panels made 349 comments about preconception care. There were approximately equal numbers of comments about clinical care issues and social and lifestyle issues. The social and lifestyle issues identified were identical to those described in Chapter 7, and are not reported again here. With respect to clinical care issues, health professionals did not take the opportunity to give preconception advice, including advice about contraception and folic acid, for 43% of women with suboptimal preconception care (table 8.2). There were concerns about screening and management of diabetes complications for nearly a tenth of the women.

Table 8.2

Panel comments on suboptimal preconception care in women with pre-existing diabetes (table contains information following categorisation of free text)

| | Women assessed to have suboptimal preconception care | | | |
| | Good pregnancy outcome (N=80) | | Poor pregnancy outcome (N=116) | |
	No. of comments	% of women	No. of comments	% of women
*Total comments**	*51*		*88*	
Suboptimal clinical practice	47	-	74	-
Folic acid not advised or prescribed	16	20	21	18
Did not take opportunity to give preconception advice	12	15	20	17
Poor screening or management of diabetes complications	8	10	9	8
Contraception not advised	6	8	10	9
Suboptimal review of medication	1	1	8	7
Other	4	5	7	6
Communication between health professionals or between health service and woman	2	3	9	8
Miscellaneous	2	3	5	4

* There were 70 comments where the woman did not receive folic acid and 3 comments where she did not have preconception care, where it was unclear as to whether this was a clinical care or social and lifestyle issue; these comments are not included in the table. There were 137 comments on social and lifestyle issues, however these were identical to the themes underlying suboptimal preconception glycaemic control (Chapter 7) and are not described further in this report.

8.6 Glycaemic control tests and targets

Regular testing of long term glycaemic control using glycosylated haemoglobin (HbA1c) is important in order to inform the management of glycaemic control (Diabetes NSF 2001).[1] Targets for glycaemic control should be set and discussed with women before pregnancy, so that they can take control of managing their diabetes more effectively.

8.6.1 Enquiry findings

Just over half (58%, 218/379) of women in the enquiry (54% of 192 cases and 62% of 187 controls) were reported to have had a test of glycaemic control in the 12 months before pregnancy. This compares favourably with the 37% reported for the full cohort of 3808 diabetic pregnancies.[2] This may be because the enquiry data related to 12 months before conception rather than just 6 months as for the full cohort, and may also be due to the fact that information for the full cohort was dependent upon medical records at secondary care, while in the enquiry module the general practitioner and adult diabetes service were also approached for information.

Sixteen percent of 379 women did not have a glycaemic control test in the year before pregnancy, and for more than a quarter (27%, 101/379) of women there was no documentation available.

There was evidence that targets for glycaemic control had been set before pregnancy for only 28% of 369 women (24% of 188 cases and 32% of 181 controls); for 52% of women, there was no documentation in the medical records (either at primary or secondary care) about targets.

8.7 Panel assessment of glycaemic control before pregnancy

The enquiry panels assessed that 79% of 354 women with available documentation (88% of 187 cases and 69% of 167 controls) had suboptimal glycaemic control before pregnancy. Women who had suboptimal preconception glycaemic control were more likely to go on to have a poor pregnancy outcome (OR 3.89, 95% CI 2.15 - 7.02, adjusted for maternal age and deprivation, see Chapter 6).

8.7.1 Panel comments on suboptimal preconception glycaemic control

The majority of enquiry panel comments related to social and lifestyle issues, and these are described in Chapter 7. However, there were 48 comments about clinical care (table 8.3). The main concerns about clinical practice were a lack of timely clinical input by health professionals to improve glycaemic control, and also concerns that the insulin regime advised was inadequate to achieve tighter control. Suboptimal communication referred mainly to poor follow-up of non-attenders and women who had lost contact with the health service.

Table 8.3

Panel comments about clinical care issues related to suboptimal preconception glycaemic control (table contains information following categorisation of free text)

	Women assessed to have suboptimal preconception glycaemic control			
	Good pregnancy outcome (N=115)		Poor pregnancy outcome (N=165)	
	No. of comments	% of women	No. of comments	% of women
Total comments*†	*20*		*28*	
Suboptimal clinical practice	15	13	11	7
Suboptimal communication	5	4	16	10
Miscellaneous	0	0	1	1

* There were 81 comments where the issues were not described by panels and 18 comments where there was a lack of preconception care with the reason being unclear to panels; these comments are not included in this table.

† 187 comments were made on social and lifestyle issues; these are described in Chapter 7.

8.8 Conclusions

Prior to pregnancy, clinical support and information for women appeared to be poor:

- Just over half of women had a retinal examination and a renal function test in the 12 months before pregnancy.

- Only a quarter of women had evidence of glycaemic control targets being set and just over half had documented evidence of a discussion about glycaemic control in the 12 months prior to pregnancy.

- Less than half of women had documented evidence that diet, contraception, or diabetes complications had been discussed in the 12 months before pregnancy.

- Less than half of women were documented to be informed about fetal risks, the increased chance of induction of labour and the possibility of caesarean delivery.

- Documentation of pre-pregnancy counselling was poor.

Enquiry panels found that health professionals often missed the opportunity to provide pre-pregnancy counselling, and did not appear to advise about or prescribe folic acid or contraception before pregnancy. There were also concerns about a lack of timely input by the diabetes team and whether insulin regimes in the preconception period were appropriate to achieve tight glycaemic control.

These findings suggest that the majority of women with diabetes are not having effective annual diabetes reviews, and that the maternity component of preconception care (contraception, folic acid, information about the impact of diabetes on pregnancy) is missing for many women.

Preconception care:

- 'No folic acid prescribed or started, even though the pregnancy was planned and the woman was having treatment to aid fertility.'
- 'Only one pre-pregnancy appointment, no folate, no smoking advice, or advice about contraception' .
- 'No retinal screening. Planned pregnancy no adequate monitoring. Inadequate care by GP and primary care. Low dose folic acid.'
- 'Despite 16 visits no evidence of input from a consultant physician.'
- 'No retinal checks or discussion of diabetes control.'
- 'Evidence of retinopathy & microalbuminuria present but not given an appointment for one year. Woman's attendance and compliance was poor, but no documentation of a definite plan. ACE inhibitor prescribed. Not a planned pregnancy - folic acid not given.'
- 'No folic acid. Type 2 diabetes on metformin. ACE inhibitor (Perindopril) not stopped. BMI 52. No recorded thyroid function test, on thyroxine for hypothyroidism 1 year.'

Glycaemic control:

- 'HbA1c>8 Panel felt: Health care professionals could have done more to help patient to reduce HbA1c. Panel felt that this woman may have needed insulin. Patient did no follow diet.'
- 'HBA1c 10.2. Sought pre-pregnancy advice. Documented advice by consultant physician to GP to change insulin, this was not acted upon.'
- 'Pre-pregnancy HbA1c was 14.4% but mother not reviewed for 6 weeks, HbA1c then 13.8%. Inappropriate small doses of insulin'
- 'HBA1c 7.7%. Twice daily insulin regime that was not adequate. No evidence of pre-pregnancy planning. Physician quotes that control good, this may have misled woman re pregnancy risks. Overcautious to avoid hypos'

8.9 Recommendations

Clinical

1. Commissioners of services must ensure that all women with diabetes are provided with specialist preconception services, with access to all members of the specialist multidisciplinary team. As a minimum, these services should include:
   - Clear signposting to different aspects of care
   - Diet and lifestyle advice
   - Provision of appropriate contraception
   - Higher dose folic acid supplementation
   - Smoking cessation support
   - Assessment and management of diabetes complications

- Setting of glycaemic control targets and regular discussion of results of self-monitoring, to enable the woman to achieve control that is as near to normal as possible before conception
- Discussion of diabetes pregnancy risks and expected management strategies
- Clear documentation of care and counselling, ideally using a standard template.

Audit and research

2. Preconception services should be audited to ensure that minimum standards are being met.

References

1. *National Service Framework for Diabetes (England) Standards.* Department of Health. The Stationery Office: London: 2001.
2. *Confidential Enquiry into Maternal and Child Health. Pregnancy in women with type 1 and type 2 diabetes in 2002-03, England, Wales and Northern Ireland.* CEMACH: London; 2005.
3. Macintosh M, Fleming K, Bailey J, Doyle P, Modder J, Acolet D, et al. *Perinatal mortality and congenital anomalies in babies of women with type 1 or type 2 diabetes in England, Wales and Northern Ireland: population based study.* BMJ, 22 Jul 2006: 333 (7560):177.
4. *Pregnancy outcomes in the Diabetes Complications Trial.* The Diabetes Control and Complications Trial Research Group. Am J Obstet Gynecol; 1996; 174: 1343-53.
5. Lumley J, Watson L, Watson M, Bower C. Cochrane Pregnancy and Childbirth Group. *Periconceptional supplementation with folate and/or multivitamins for preventing neural tube defects.* Cochrane Database of Systematic Reviews. 2006, 3.
6. *Confidential Enquiry into Maternal and Child Health. Survey of maternity services for women with type 1 and type 2 diabetes in 2002-03, England, Wales and Northern Ireland.* CEMACH: London; 2005.

Commentary

Sue Roberts
National Clinical Director for Diabetes
Consultant Diabetes Physician, North Tyneside General Hospital

This chapter paints a disturbing picture of a lack of diabetes preconception care services across England, Wales and Northern Ireland, and a lack of knowledge both on the part of healthcare professionals and women with diabetes, about the importance of preconception care. The evidence indicates that preconception care is vital in trying to ensure that both mothers and babies have as safe and healthy a pregnancy and birth as possible. The findings in this report suggest that when there is suboptimal preconception care, pregnancy outcomes can be devastating for the mother-to-be and her baby.

Adult diabetes services and primary care professionals are often in contact with women prior to pregnancy, and therefore have a real responsibility to provide relevant information and monitoring, both in the immediate pre-pregnancy period and as part of women's routine care. In the current situation, many women are missing out on information and monitoring as part of their routine care on a year by year basis.

Apart from the explanation of pregnancy risks and the need to maintain good glycaemic control, some drugs which may be prescribed for women with type 2 diabetes, such as ACE inhibitors, are harmful in pregnancy. This emphasis on informing women of the risks and the preventive actions they can take, means that diabetes services for women of child bearing age should be planned in a slightly different way to other diabetes services. This is supported by the recently developed diabetes workforce competencies[c] that specifically address the needs of women of child bearing age with diabetes, as well as those actively seeking to become pregnant, and those who are already pregnant.

The current absence of structured preconception care needs to be set within the context of the increasing number of women of child bearing age with diabetes – mainly type 2 diabetes. This rise has been fuelled by a number of factors, including the increasing obesity of the general population, changing ethnic demographics and reducing levels of exercise and fitness. An additional factor is that women from ethnic minority groups with an increased risk of type 2 diabetes, tend to have larger families. The General Household Survey 1988-2001[d] found that women of Bangladeshi origin tended on average to have families twice as large as the White population.

The Diabetes National Service Framework (NSF) recommends that all diabetes services should be effectively planned, but it is clear that this is currently not the case for the majority of local services across the country, either for routine or preconception care. While pregnancy in women with diabetes used to be considered a specialist activity, there is now a critical need for services to be planned jointly in primary as well as secondary care in order to achieve integrated models of preconception and pregnancy care. This is an immense challenge, and diabetes networks have a crucial role in supporting this planning and commissioning process by enabling each of the stakeholders to identify needs and priorities.

Although it may be difficult to accept, we must understand that pregnancy for women with diabetes will always be high risk. However, it is our responsibility to discover new ways of working with women that will reduce the risks and ensure the best possible outcomes, both for them and their babies.

[c] Skills for Health, Diabetes Workforce Competencies, 2006.

[d] Sources: Census 2001, Office for National Statistics; General Register Office for Scotland.

9. Clinical care issues: pregnancy

> **Learning points**
>
> - Suboptimal glycaemic control during pregnancy was associated with poor pregnancy outcome. The main clinical issues identified were failure to change insulin regimes to achieve good glycaemic control, and a non-responsive local strategy of diabetes antenatal care.
>
> - Suboptimal maternity care and diabetes care (excluding glycaemic control) during pregnancy was associated with poor pregnancy outcome. Underlying issues included suboptimal fetal and maternal surveillance and suboptimal monitoring of diabetes complications.
>
> - For babies with antenatal evidence of macrosomia, suboptimal antenatal fetal surveillance was associated with poor pregnancy outcome, with the main issues being lack of timely follow up and poor interpretation of ultrasound scans.
>
> - Women who had a poor pregnancy outcome were more likely not to receive postnatal contraceptive advice and more likely to have suboptimal postnatal diabetes care.

9.1 Introduction

During pregnancy, there are often rapid changes in glycaemic control due to increasing insulin resistance. Suboptimal glycaemic control has been associated with fetal congenital anomaly,[1] an increased risk of miscarriage[2] and fetal macrosomia;[3] and there may also be placental insufficiency (particularly associated with nephropathy) resulting in fetal growth restriction. Women themselves may have complications including hypoglycaemia, retinopathy, nephropathy, diabetic ketoacidosis and pre-eclampsia. Clinicians and health services have an important role in building relationships with women before and during pregnancy, empowering them to manage their diabetes, and providing effective maternal and fetal surveillance.

9.2 Glycaemic control during pregnancy, labour and delivery

Tight glycaemic control during pregnancy is one of the main principles of management for women with pre-existing diabetes. During labour and delivery, good glycaemic control should be maintained to reduce the risk of neonatal hypoglycaemia.[4]

The 2005 CEMACH report[5] on pregnant women with pre-existing diabetes found that although approximately three quarters of 2732 women had a glycosylated haemoglobin test (HbA1c) performed during the first trimester of pregnancy, just over a third of these women achieved an HbA1c value less than 7%. This improved in the second and third trimesters, with two thirds of women with an HbA1c test achieving a result less than 7%.

9.2.1 Enquiry findings

Enquiry panels assessed that the majority of women in the enquiry had suboptimal glycaemic control during pregnancy (84% of 204 cases and 61% of 192 controls in the first trimester; 71% of 205 cases and 37% of 209 controls after the first trimester). Suboptimal glycaemic control at any time during pregnancy was associated with poor pregnancy outcome (OR 3.4, 95% CI 2.1 - 5.7 in first trimester and OR 5.2, 95% CI 3.3 - 8.2 after first trimester, both ORs adjusted for maternal age and deprivation, see Chapter 0).

Fifty percent (176/354) of women (49% of 162 cases, 48% of 202 controls) with ongoing pregnancies after 24 weeks were assessed by panels to have suboptimal glycaemic control during labour and/or delivery.

9.2.2 Panel comments on suboptimal glycaemic control during pregnancy

The majority of panel comments related to social and lifestyle issues and these are described in Chapter 7. However, there were 178 panel comments made on clinical care issues, with the main concern being suboptimal clinical practice (table 9.1). This included failure to change insulin regimes to achieve good glycaemic control, and a non-responsive local strategy of diabetes antenatal care, including lack of support, failure to follow up women, and poor integration of the care provided by different disciplines. Problems within the diabetes multidisciplinary team included lack of involvement of consultant obstetricians or diabetes physicians, and lack of dietetic input.

Table 9.1

Panel comments on suboptimal glycaemic control during pregnancy in women with type 1 and type 2 diabetes (table contains information following categorisation of free text)

	Women assessed to have suboptimal glycaemic control in 1st trimester				Women assessed to have suboptimal glycaemic control after 1st trimester			
	Good pregnancy outcome (N=118)		Poor pregnancy outcome (N=171)		Good pregnancy outcome (N=76)		Poor pregnancy outcome (N=146)	
	No. of comments	% of women	No. of comments	% of women	No. of comments	% of women	No. of comments	% of women
*Total comments**	*34*	-	*46*		*35*	-	*63*	
Suboptimal clinical practice	30	-	32	-	27	-	47	-
Failure to change insulin regime	13	11	9	5	11	14	18	12
Non-responsive local strategy of diabetes antenatal care	7	6	9	5	9	12	15	10
Problems within diabetes multidisciplinary team	8	7	4	2	6	8	10	7
Lack of preconception care	2	2	5	3	0	-	2	1
Inappropriate management (other than insulin)	0	-	4	2	1	1	2	1
Did not follow guideline	0	-	1	1	0	-	0	-
Poor documentation / communication	4	3	14	8	8	11	16	11

* 248 comments were made on social and lifestyle issues. In 198 comments, panels did not describe the specific issue underlying suboptimal glycaemic control.

9.2.3 Panel comments on suboptimal glycaemic control during labour and delivery

The guidance given to enquiry panels was that optimal glycaemic control during labour and delivery referred to blood glucose values between 3.5 – 8 mmols/l, although this was not prescriptive. The target range recommended by Diabetes UK for labour and delivery is 4– 6 mmol/l[6] and the Diabetes NSF recommends tight blood glucose control during labour.[7]

Panels made 211 comments for 176 women about suboptimal glycaemic control during labour and delivery. The main issue identified was suboptimal clinical practice, particularly concerns about inadequate intravenous insulin/dextrose regimes, delays in commencing intravenous regimes and the subsequent management of those regimes (table 9.2).

Table 9.2

Panel comments on suboptimal glycaemic control during labour and delivery (table contains information following categorisation of free text)

	Women assessed to have suboptimal glycaemic control during labour and delivery			
	Good pregnancy outcome n=96		Poor pregnancy outcome n=80	
	No. of comments	% of women	No. of comments	% of women
*Total comments**	98	-	70	-
Suboptimal clinical practice	90	-	62	-
Inappropriate intravenous insulin/ dextrose regime	26	27	8	11
Delay in starting intravenous insulin/ dextrose regime	19	19	14	20
Poor management of sliding scale	17	17	17	24
Suboptimal blood glucose monitoring	15	15	10	14
Hypoglycaemia due to clinical practice	2	2	4	6
Poor management of hypoglycaemia	4	4	2	3
Other clinical practice issues	7	7	7	10
Communication issues	4	4	6	9
Resource issues	2	2	0	0
Patient issues	2	2	2	3

* The underlying issues were not described in 43 comments made by panels.

9.3 Glycaemic control targets

It is important that women should be informed of what short and long term glycaemic control targets they are trying to achieve, to enable them to optimise their control.

9.3.1 Enquiry findings

Target ranges for glycaemic control were documented in the medical records or local hospital guidelines for just over half of women during pregnancy (53%, 232/440 of women in the first trimester and 54%, 239/441 of women after the first trimester up to labour and delivery). This improved during labour and delivery, with 79% of the 384 women delivering after 24 weeks having a target range documented.

When a target range was present during pregnancy, there was evidence that this had been communicated to the woman for only 48% of the 232 women in the first trimester and 51% of the 239 women after the first trimester.

9.4 Diabetes care - monitoring for diabetes complications

In addition to achieving good glycaemic control during pregnancy, women with diabetes also need ongoing monitoring and treatment for diabetes complications. There may be development of new retinopathy or deterioration of pre-existing retinopathy during pregnancy,[8] and women should have a full retinal assessment during the first trimester,[7] with prompt referral to an ophthalmologist if an abnormality is found.

Women with diabetes nephropathy are at increased risk of hypertensive disease of pregnancy, adverse fetal outcomes, and progressive deterioration of renal disease.[9-11] Enquiry panels were not provided with an explicit standard of monitoring for nephropathy, but were provided with the guidance that appropriate monitoring included testing for microalbuminuria (incipient nephropathy), protein dipstick testing of urine or serum creatinine.

9.4.1 Enquiry findings

Just over half of women (59%, 258/441), had a retinal assessment documented during the first trimester or at the first booking visit. Only 55% of these 258 assessments were recorded to have been done through dilated pupils; for 40% of women, details about the retinal assessment procedure were not documented. Seventy eight percent (343/441) of women were monitored for signs of nephropathy. Lack of monitoring for nephropathy was associated with poor pregnancy outcome (OR 1.9, 95% CI 1.1 - 3.3, adjusted for maternal age and deprivation, see Chapter 6). However, in the additional case control analysis (see Appendices C, D and E), lack of monitoring for nephropathy was associated only with fetal congenital anomaly and not with fetal or neonatal death after 20 weeks gestation, and is therefore unlikely to have been causative for poor pregnancy outcome. Nephropathy itself was not associated with poor pregnancy outcome.

Enquiry panels assessed that 60% (264/440) of women (72% of 204 cases and 58% of 204 controls) had suboptimal diabetes care (care other than glycaemic control management) during pregnancy. These women were more likely to have a poor pregnancy outcome (OR 1.7, 95% CI 1.1 - 2.6, adjusted for maternal age and deprivation, see Chapter 6). Additional case-control analysis (see Appendices C, D and E) showed an association with fetal or neonatal death from 20 weeks gestation and not with fetal congenital anomaly.

9.4.2 Panel comments on suboptimal diabetes care in pregnancy

Panels made 432 comments for 264 women about suboptimal diabetes care in pregnancy, with the majority of these being concerns about suboptimal clinical practice (table 9.3).

Table 9.3

Panel comments on suboptimal diabetes care (excluding glycaemic control) in pregnancy (table contains information following categorisation of free text)

	Women assessed to have suboptimal diabetes care in pregnancy			
	Good pregnancy outcome n=118		Poor pregnancy outcome n=146	
	No. of comments	% of women	No. of comments	% of women
*Total comments**	*174*	-	*224*	-
Suboptimal clinical practice	**159**		**196**	
Lack of /suboptimal retinal screening/ management	72	61	71	49
Suboptimal renal function monitoring/ management	38	32	49	34
Lack of multidisciplinary involvement	25	21	31	21
Lack of senior input	2	2	7	5
Poor management of glycaemic control during steroid administration	1	1	1	1
Suboptimal management of pre-pregnancy medication	0	0	2	1
Suboptimal management of other complications e.g. proteinuria +/-BP, ketonuria	6	5	12	8
Infrequent clinic appointments	2	2	9	6
Other	13	11	14	10
Communication issues	**5**	**4**	**9**	**6**
Patient factors	**10**	**8**	**19**	**13**

* 34 comments were about social and lifestyle issues.

9.5 Antenatal fetal surveillance

Careful fetal surveillance is important in diabetic pregnancy, including serial ultrasound scans for fetal growth during the third trimester and consideration of cardiotocograph monitoring from 36 weeks.[7] Enquiry panels assessed that fetal surveillance was suboptimal for 20% of 37 babies with antenatal evidence of fetal growth restriction and for 45% of 129 babies with antenatal evidence of macrosomia (defined for panel enquiries as fetal size >90th centile). For babies with antenatal evidence of macrosomia, suboptimal fetal surveillance was associated with poor pregnancy outcome (OR 5.3, 95% CI 2.4 -12.0, adjusted for maternal age and deprivation, see Chapter 6). Additional case-control analysis (see Appendices C, D and E) showed an association with fetal or neonatal death after 20 weeks gestation and not with fetal congenital anomaly.

9.5.1 Panel comments on suboptimal antenatal fetal surveillance

Panels made 89 comments for 65 women about suboptimal antenatal fetal surveillance. The main issue for both macrosomic and growth restricted babies was a lack of timely follow-up (table 9.4). For macrosomic babies, there were also concerns about poor interpretation of ultrasound scans and about actions taken as a response to tests.

Table 9.4

Panel comments on suboptimal antenatal fetal surveillance in women with pre-existing diabetes (table contains information following categorisation of free text)

	Babies assessed to have suboptimal antenatal fetal surveillance			
	Growth restricte babies (N=7)		Macrosomic babies (N=58)	
	No. of comments	% of babies	No. of comments	% of babies
*Total comments**	8	-	74	-
Suboptimal clinical practice	8	-	73	
Lack of timely follow-up	6	86	47	81
Should have had additional investigations	0	14	2	3
Poor interpretation of surveillance	1	14	11	19
Incorrect actions taken	1	14	11	19
Poor standard of investigative procedure	0	-	2	3
Poor communication	0	-	1	2

* There were 4 comments where the issues were not described by panels, and 3 comments about social and lifestyle issues.

9.6 Management of antenatal steroid administration

Women with pre-existing diabetes have a higher preterm delivery and spontaneous preterm labour rate compared to the general maternity population.[5] Women who are at risk of preterm delivery and require prophylactic antenatal steroids need careful management of glycaemic control to minimise the risk of diabetic ketoacidosis, and it is recommended that additional insulin should be given during this time.[6,7]

9.6.1 Management of glycaemic control with antenatal steroids

In the 2005 CEMACH study, 70% of women delivering a live born baby before 34 weeks received prophylactic steroids.[5]

In the enquiry, 56 women delivering before 34 weeks gestation received antenatal steroids. The majority of these women (68%, 38/56), were commenced on an intravenous insulin and dextrose infusion during treatment. However, a tenth of women did not have any change in glycaemic control management despite having been given antenatal steroids (table 9.5).

Table 9.5	
Management of glycaemic control during antenatal steroid administration in women with diabetes delivering before 34 weeks gestation	
Management of glycaemic control with antenatal steroid administration	**No. of women receiving corticosteroids n(%) (N=56)**
No change from prior management	6 (11)
Increased checking of blood glucose only	3 (5)
Subcutaneous insulin regime changed*	3 (5)
Intravenous insulin and dextrose infusion started*	38 (68)
Information not available	6 (11)

* Women who had a change in subcutaneous insulin regime or who started intravenous insulin and dextrose infusion, also had increased checking of blood glucose.

9.7 Discussion of mode and timing of delivery

Women with pre-existing diabetes have high rates of obstetric intervention, with a 39% induction of labour rate and a 67% caesarean section rate.[5] It is important that women should be involved in the decision-making process regarding mode and timing of delivery.

9.7.1 Enquiry findings

A discussion about mode and timing of delivery was documented in the medical records for 86% (329/384) of women who delivered after 24+0 weeks gestation. The first discussion occurred at a median of 35 weeks (range 5 - 40 weeks). A lack of discussion of mode and timing of delivery was associated with poor pregnancy outcome (OR 4.0, 95% CI 1.2 - 12.7, adjusted for maternal age and deprivation, see Chapter 6). Additional case-control analysis (see Appendices C, D and E) showed an association with fetal or neonatal death from 20 weeks gestation but not with fetal congenital anomaly. However, women who did not have a documented discussion delivered at an earlier gestation than women who had evidence of a discussion (median gestation at delivery 35 weeks versus 37 weeks), and there may therefore have been other factors contributing to poor outcome.

9.8 Maternity care during pregnancy, labour and delivery

Women with pre-existing diabetes have an increased risk of fetal and maternal complications and it is important that there is ongoing fetal and maternal surveillance throughout pregnancy, labour and delivery to identify and manage any risks.

Enquiry panels assessed that maternity care during pregnancy was suboptimal for 51% of 430 women (58% of 215 cases and 44% of 215 controls), and these women were more likely to have a poor pregnancy outcome (OR 1.9, 95% CI 1.2 - 2.8, adjusted for maternal age and deprivation, see Chapter 6). Additional case-control analysis (see Appendices C, D and E) showed an association with fetal or neonatal death from 20 weeks gestation but not with fetal congenital anomaly.

During labour and delivery, the majority of women were assessed to have optimal maternity care. Care was assessed to be suboptimal for 35% of 382 women , with no association between suboptimal care and pregnancy outcome (see Chapter 6).

9.8.1 Panel comments on suboptimal maternity care during pregnancy

Panels made 378 comments for 228 women, with nearly all of these being about clinical care issues. The two largest categories related to suboptimal fetal surveillance (ultrasound monitoring of fetal growth and fetal heart rate monitoring) and management of maternal risks. Problems with the antenatal diabetes multidisciplinary team, communication and the level of seniority of obstetric staff involved in the woman's care were also noted (table 9.6).

Table 9.6

Panel comments on suboptimal maternity care during pregnancy for women with pre-existing diabetes (table contains information following categorisation of free text)

| | Women assessed to have suboptimal maternity care during pregnancy | | | |
| | Good pregnancy outcome (N–95) | | Poor pregnancy outcome (N=125) | |
	No. of comments	% of women	No. of comments	% of women
Total comments[^]	*147*	-	*209*	-
Suboptimal clinical practice	**141**	-	**178**	-
Fetal surveillance	47	49	58	46
Management of maternal risks	29	31	39	31
Problem with the multidisciplinary team	17	18	28	22
Need for more senior obstetrician input	11	12	24	19
Mode and timing of delivery	20	21	10	8
No plan of care	7	7	15	12
Steroids not given/full course not completed	4	4	2	2
Other	6	6	2	2
Communication	**6**	**6**	**31**	**25**

* 22 comments were made about social and lifestyle issues; these comments are not included in this table.

9.8.2 Panel comments on suboptimal maternity care during labour and delivery

Enquiry panels made 245 comments for 150 women. The most frequent issues noted were poor management of maternal risks, inappropriate decisions relating to delivery and inadequate fetal surveillance during labour or delay in acting on signs of fetal compromise (table 9.7).

Table 9.7

Panel comments on suboptimal maternity care during labour and delivery

| | Women assessed to have suboptimal maternity care during labour and delivery | | | |
| | Good pregnancy outcome (N=72) | | Poor pregnancy outcome (N=78) | |
	No. of comments	% of women	No. of comments	% of women
*Total comments**	*123*	-	*120*	-
Suboptimal clinical practice	**90**	-	**96**	-
Poor management of maternal risks	19	26	28	36
Inappropriate decisions relating to delivery[†]	26	36	14	18
Inadequate fetal surveillance/delay in acting on evidence of fetal compromise	20	28	18	23
Insufficient senior obstetric input	8	11	12	15
Poor management of second stage	7	10	12	15
Poor management of induction/first stage of labour	8	11	8	10
No plan of management	2	3	4	5
Communication	**14**	**19**	**13**	**17**
Anaesthetic issues	**4**	**6**	**3**	**4**
Resource	**3**	**4**	**1**	**1**
Other	**12**	**17**	**7**	**9**

* 2 comments were made about social and lifestyle issues; these comments are not included in this table.

† includes inappropriate decision to expedite delivery and inappropriate mode of delivery.

9.9 Postnatal care

Women with diabetes will usually deliver in a consultant-led unit and be cared for by maternity staff. Good lines of communication between maternity and diabetes teams are therefore important, and maternity staff should have easy access to expert advice about glycaemic control. A clear written plan for diabetes management in the woman's medical records is important to help maternity staff provide appropriate care.

Clinicians should take the opportunity to provide information and advice about contraception and the importance of planned pregnancy before the woman is discharged from hospital. Women should have a follow up diabetes appointment after discharge from hospital to discuss ongoing management of glycaemic control and continue with other aspects of their diabetes care.

9.9.1 Enquiry findings

The majority of women, (81%, 312/383) delivering after 24 weeks gestation had a documented plan for post delivery diabetes management. Seventy three percent (280/383) of women had a follow up diabetes appointment arranged.

Just 52% of 383 women (38% of 164 cases and 63% of 219 controls) were documented to have had contraceptive advice provided before discharge from hospital. Women who had had a poor pregnancy outcome were more likely not to receive contraceptive advice than women with a good pregnancy outcome (OR 4.2, 95% CI 2.4 - 7.4, adjusted for maternal age and deprivation, see Chapter 6)

Enquiry panels assessed that 57% of 364 women (66% of 153 cases and 50% of 211 controls) delivering after 24 weeks gestation had suboptimal postnatal diabetes care and advice. Women who had a poor pregnancy outcome were more likely to have suboptimal postnatal diabetes care (adjusted OR 1.8, 95% CI 1.2 - 2.7, adjusted for maternal age and deprivation, see Chapter 6).

9.9.2 Panel comments on suboptimal postnatal diabetes care

Panels made 267 comments for 207 women, with the majority of these being related to suboptimal clinical care. Concerns included management of glycaemic control after delivery, inadequate plans of care at discharge from hospital, lack of contact with the diabetes team and no contraceptive advice given to women (table 9.8).

Table 9.8

Panel comments about suboptimal postnatal diabetes care (table contains information following categorisation of free text)

| | Women assessed to have suboptimal postnatal diabetes care | | | |
| | Good pregnancy outcome (N=106) | | Poor pregnancy outcome (N=101) | |
	No. of comments	% of women	No. of comments	% of women
*Total comments**	*95*		*129*	
Suboptimal clinical practice	**95**	-	**129**	-
Suboptimal management of glycaemic control	40	38	31	31
Inadequate plan of care at discharge	24	23	36	36
Lack of contact with diabetes team	15	14	30	30
No contraceptive advice	14	13	29	29
Other	2	2	3	3

* There were 32 comments where the underlying issues were not described by panels, and 11 comments about social and lifestyle issues; these comments are not included in this table.

9.10 Conclusions

It is encouraging that there were a number of areas of good practice identified:

- 78% of women were monitored for nephropathy
- 79% of women had evidence of glycaemic control targets for labour and delivery
- 68% of women receiving antenatal steroids had an insulin and dextrose infusion commenced
- 86% of women had a documented discussion about timing and mode of delivery
- 65% of women had optimal maternity care during labour and delivery
- 81% of women had a written plan for post-delivery diabetes management.

However, there were a number of concerns about clinical care during pregnancy. Nearly half of women in the enquiry did not have a retinal examination during the first trimester and there were concerns about failure to change insulin regimes to achieve good glycaemic control, and a non-responsive local strategy of diabetes antenatal care. A tenth of women did not have any additional interventions to ensure good glycaemic control during antenatal steroid administration. Fetal surveillance was suboptimal for nearly half of babies with antenatal evidence of macrosomia, and this was associated with poor pregnancy outcome, specifically fetal or neonatal death from 20 weeks gestation (see Chapter 6 and Appendices C, D and E).

It is disappointing that women who had a poor pregnancy outcome were more likely to have suboptimal diabetes care after delivery and were less likely to receive contraceptive advice prior to discharge from hospital. It is recognised that clinicians are likely to need to provide more intensive counselling to women who have had a fetal loss, stillbirth or a baby born with a congenital anomaly, and discussion about contraception in this situation can be difficult. However, it is important that diabetes care is not compromised for these women, and discussion about future pregnancy preparation may help to minimise the risk of adverse pregnancy outcome in the future.

Some quotes from the panel discussions

Suboptimal glycaemic control during pregnancy:

- 'HbA1C 10.7% - should have been put on insulin.'
- 'At 36 weeks HbA1c 8.6%. Insulin was changed to QDS at 28 weeks this should have been sooner.'
- 'Fragmented Care, locum consultants. No notes from Diabetologist.'

Suboptimal glycaemic control during labour and delivery:

- 'Sliding scale not commenced until well established in labour and blood glucose high. Fixed sliding scale that did not adequately maintain blood glucose at acceptable levels.'
- 'The pump became disconnected, the 3 way tap was turned off. No one noticed for some time until her BMs went up considerably.'

Diabetes care (excluding glycaemic control):

- 'Inadequate nephropathy monitoring - no regular urine testing, only 2 dipstick urine tests. No retinal screening after 13 weeks.'
- 'Lack of evidence of holistic care, seemed to be outside multidisciplinary service, no information about diabetes nurse specialist, dietetic or community team's input, no joint clinic.'

Antenatal fetal surveillance:

- 'Noted increase in abdominal circumference with previous history of IUD and the next scan is arranged for 4 weeks. There should have been increased surveillance.'

- 'No serial growth scans performed (not in protocol either). The method of management; CTGs only, inappropriate.'
- 'Stated USS good growth - despite AC >97th centile.'

Maternity care:

- 'Given steroids as outpatient.'
- 'Significant hypertension was never treated; pre-eclampsia symptoms were not addressed.'
- 'This lady was admitted to hospital on several occasions with vomiting, but was not reviewed by the medical or diabetic team. The diagnosis of DKA was not picked up on one of her admissions.'

Postnatal care

- 'Given pre-delivery dose of insulin post delivery, despite the Registrar recording "use pre-delivery dose". The mother became hypoglycaemic.'
- 'One BM stix in 3 days, no evidence of plan of care and contraceptive advice left to GP.'

9.11 Recommendations

Clinical

1. An individualised care plan covering the pregnancy and postnatal period up to 6 weeks should be clearly documented in the notes, ideally using a standard template. The plan may require changes to be made depending on the clinical circumstances through pregnancy. As a minimum, the care plan should include:
   - Targets for glycaemic control
   - Retinal screening schedule
   - Renal screening schedule
   - Fetal surveillance
   - Plan for delivery
   - Diabetes care after delivery.
2. The care plan should be implemented from the outset of pregnancy by a multidisciplinary team present at the same time in the same clinic. As a minimum, the multidisciplinary team should include an obstetrician, diabetes physician, diabetes specialist nurse, diabetes midwife and dietitian.
3. Pregnancies with ultrasound evidence of macrosomia should have a clear management plan put in place by a consultant obstetrician. This should include timing of follow-up scans, fetal surveillance and mode and timing of delivery.
4. A care plan for postnatal management should be clearly documented in the notes for all women. As a minimum, this should include:
   - Plan for management of glycaemic control
   - Neonatal care
   - Contraception
   - Follow-up care after discharge from hospital.

Audit and research

5. Research should be carried out to investigate:
    *   the most appropriate management strategy following antenatal evidence of macrosomia in babies of women with diabetes
    *   how best to achieve optimal blood glucose control during pregnancy, labour and delivery.

References

1. Miller E, Hare JW, Cloherty JP, Dunn PJ, Gleason RE, Soeldner JS, et al. *Elevated maternal haemoglobin A1c in early pregnancy and major congenital anomalies in infants of diabetic mother.* N Engl J Med, 1981.304:1331-4.
2. Mills JL, Simpson JL, Driscoll SG, Jovanovic-Peterson L, Van Allen M, Aarons JH, Metzger B, Bieber FR, Knopp RH, Holmes LB et al. *Incidence of spontaneous abortion among normal women and insulin-dependent diabetic women whose pregnancies were identified within 21 days of conception.* N Engl J Med, 1988: 319:1617-1623.
3. Rey E, Attie C, Bonin A. *The effects of first-trimester diabetes control on the incidence of macrosomia.* Am J Obstet Gynecol, 1999; 181, 202-6.
4. Taylor R, Lee C, Kyne-Grzebalski D, Marshall SM, Davison JM. *Clinical outcomes of pregnancy in women with type 1 diabetes.* Obstet Gynecol, 2002; 99, 537 – 41.
5. *Confidential Enquiry into Maternal and Child Health. Pregnancy in women with type 1 and type 2 diabetes in 2002-03, England, Wales and Northern Ireland.* CEMACH: London; 2005.
6. *Recommendations for the management of pregnant women with diabetes (including gestational diabetes).* Diabetes UK Care Recommendation. Updated June 2005.
7. *National Service Framework for Diabetes (England) Standards.* Department of Health. The Stationery Office: London; 2001.
8. Sheth BP. *Does pregnancy accelerate the rate of progression of diabetic retinopathy?* Current Diabetes Reports, Aug 2002: 2(4):327-30.
9. Duckitt K, Harrington D. *Risk factors for pre-eclampsia at antenatal booking: systematic review of controlled studies.* BMJ, 12 Mar 2005: 330(7491):565.
10. Fischer MJ, Lehnerz SD, Hebert JR, Parikh CR. *Kidney disease is an independent risk factor for adverse fetal and maternal outcomes in pregnancy.* American Journal of Kidney Diseases. Mar 2004: 43(3):415-23.
11. Irfan S, Arain TM, Shaukat A, Shahid A. *Effect of pregnancy on diabetic nephropathy and retinopathy.* J Coll Physicians Surg Pak: Feb 2004: 14(2):75-8.

Commentary

Stephen Walkinshaw
Chair, CEMACH Diabetes Professional Advisory Group
Consultant Obstetrician, Liverpool Women's Hospital, Liverpool

Although there are many areas of good clinical practice during pregnancy for women with diabetes, this chapter has highlighted some aspects of diabetes and maternity care that are less impressive.

The panel enquiries, which are in essence a detailed peer review of clinical care, have identified a number of underlying issues which may help multidisciplinary teams to work towards improving care and outcomes.

It is surprising that barely half of women in the enquiry had optimal glycaemic control after the first trimester. Some of the underlying issues included poor integration of care, failure to follow up women and failure to change insulin regimens to enable optimal glycaemic control. It should be feasible to address these issues within the organisation of multidisciplinary clinics without significant additional resource. Similarly, improving the setting of blood glucose targets, retinal and renal screening and more senior involvement should be feasible within existing local frameworks of care, though maintaining continuous senior input at the clinic may be a challenge.

Women with diabetes are a 'captive' group during labour and delivery, and it cannot be acceptable that a large number were considered to have suboptimal glycaemic control during this time, especially given the knowledge that the level of glycaemic control during labour influences the risk of neonatal hypoglycaemia. Panels noted delays in starting intravenous insulin, and inadequate dose regimens, which when taken together with panels' concerns about local guidelines in Chapter 10, suggests that the organisation of diabetes care on the labour ward needs improvement. Multidisciplinary teams need to consider how they can continue the high level of antenatal specialist involvement through to the labour ward, and how they can provide clear written guidance and practical training for non specialist staff.

Suboptimal maternity care during pregnancy, which was present in half of women in the enquiry, was associated with a two to threefold increase in the risk of losing a baby after 20 weeks. For babies with evidence of macrosomia, suboptimal fetal surveillance was strongly associated with an increased risk of death after 20 weeks gestation. The main underlying issues identified were poor antenatal fetal surveillance, poor management of maternal risks, and inappropriate decisions about mode and timing of delivery.

Though there is a relatively small evidence base for fetal surveillance in diabetic pregnancy, most women with diabetes have regular ultrasound scans and some form of fetal well-being monitoring. There is, however, little point in any form of surveillance if no or inadequate action is taken in response to the results. It suggests that such surveillance is carried out 'routinely' in many cases without detailed consideration of the possible impact on the fetus, and perhaps echoes the panels' comments about lack of senior input. Similarly, it may be that all women with diabetes are regarded as high risk without any stratification within the group, leading to poor management of individual risks and a blanket policy on mode and timing of delivery. Obstetric and midwifery members of the multidisciplinary team need to consider what tests and interventions are actually needed, and what these mean to the individual pregnancy and not for diabetic pregnancy in general. The NICE guidelines on diabetes in pregnancy, currently under development, may give some direction to these discussions.

From the panels' comments on postnatal care, it does appear that the diabetes team is not as closely involved with the woman's care after birth as before, even though 4 out of 5 women had a documented plan. Delivery of consistent quality in postnatal care is a problem outwith pregnancy in women with diabetes, and this difficult service issue will be a challenge to improve.

10. Clinical governance

10.1 Introduction

Providing a high standard of clinical care is a central tenet of clinical governance. This needs to be supported by efficient referral pathways, multidisciplinary working, good documentation, evidence-based guidelines and clear lines of communication between health professionals and between health professionals and patients. The Clinical Negligence Scheme for Trusts (CNST), administered by the NHS Litigation Authority (NHSLA), has defined minimum standards for maternity units in all these areas. This chapter examines some of the issues identified by panels for women with type 1 and type 2 diabetes using maternity services.

10.2 Access to maternity care

Women with pre-existing diabetes should be referred promptly from primary care to the diabetes specialist team as soon as pregnancy is confirmed[1], for review of glycaemic control, assessment for diabetes complications and a dating first trimester ultrasound scan. It is encouraging that women in the enquiry had their first contact with a health professional at a median of 6+6 weeks, and their first hospital appointment at 8+3 weeks.

10.3 Multidisciplinary working

Women with pre-existing diabetes require the clinical expertise of a number of different professionals during pregnancy. The Diabetes NSF recommends that antenatal care should be provided by a full multidisciplinary team comprising an obstetrician, diabetes physician, diabetes specialist nurse, midwife and dietitian.[1] In the CEMACH survey of diabetes maternity services[2], 63% of maternity units in England, Wales and Northern Ireland reported a full multidisciplinary team, and there had been an increase in specialist staff compared with the last national survey 8 years previously.[3] In particular, the availability of a dietitian in the antenatal clinic had doubled from 40% to 88% of units and the availability of a midwife specialist had tripled from 25% to 77% of units.

10.3.1 Enquiry findings

Seventy five percent (329/441) of women in the enquiry were reported to have care provided in a combined clinic. However, only 22% of 441 women were reported to have had all members of the multidisciplinary team involved in their care. The professionals most likely not to have been involved were the midwife and the dietitian (for 54% and 53% of 441 women respectively). This is surprising in view of the findings of the previous CEMACH survey. A possible reason is that women were not easily able to access dietitians and midwives even though they were members of the multidisciplinary team, perhaps due to patterns of working within the antenatal clinic. However, it is also possible that there were panel variations in interpretation of the term 'midwife with special interest in diabetes' which was used in the enquiry pro forma.

10.4 Documentation

Clear documentation of care given and plans of management enables different clinicians to effectively follow up individual women. The CNST 'Health Record' standard states that a woman's health record should provide a complete and contemporaneous record of her treatment and related features.[4]

10.4.1 Enquiry findings

Enquiry panels' consensus was that there were deficiencies in the standard of 44% of 436 obstetric notes and 51% of 439 diabetes notes.

For both diabetes and obstetric notes, the main issue identified for 55% and 61% of women respectively where deficiencies were identified, was poor documentation of what care had been given and the plan of care (table 10.1). In many instances diabetes information was so scanty that panels questioned whether the diabetes notes had been written elsewhere. In a fifth of cases there were concerns that the design of the notes was not fit for purpose for antenatal care of a woman with diabetes.

Table 10.1

Panel comments on deficiencies in obstetric and diabetes notes (table contains information following categorisation of free text)

	Obstetric notes (N=192)		Diabetes notes (N=224)	
	No. of comments*	% of notes	No. of comments	% of notes
*Total comments**	*210*		*236*	
Poor documentation of care given or care plans	105	55	136	61
Poor design of notes	40	21	53	24
Missing notes or CTGs	30	16	40	18
Fetal growth not plotted on scans	14	7	-	-
Grade of staff not recorded	8	4	3	1
Illegible writing	9	5	3	1
Date/time not recorded	4	2	1	0

* In 1 panel comment, the issue was not specified.

10.5 Maternity unit guidelines

CNST emphasises the importance of evidence-based, referenced, multidisciplinary guidelines which are easily accessible to the health professionals providing care.[4] For each woman in the enquiry, panels were asked to review the local maternity unit's diabetes guideline (contemporaneous for 2002-2003) when these had been provided by the unit. An individual unit's guideline may have been reviewed more than once by panels, and the results are therefore presented as the proportion of women to whom any concerns related.

Enquiry panels had concerns about local maternity units' diabetes guidelines for nearly three quarters (72%) of 386 women where unit guidelines were available.

10.5.1 Panel comments on maternity unit diabetes guidelines

Panels made 386 comments about the local diabetes guidelines for 278 women. The two most frequent issues cited were no antenatal guidelines and lack of clarity or insufficient detail (table 10.2). For nearly a quarter of the women, the panels' view was that intravenous insulin regimes for labour were inadequate, and for approximately a fifth of the women the guideline did not include blood glucose targets. There was considered to be wrong or inappropriate advice in the guidelines for more than a tenth of women assessed to have suboptimal local guidelines.

Table 10.2 Panel comments on suboptimal maternity unit diabetes guidelines (table contains information following categorisation of free text)		
	Number of women with suboptimal local guidelines (N=278)	
	No. of comments	% of women
*Total comments**	*386*	-
No antenatal guideline	80	29
Not enough detail/not clear	70	25
Inadequate intravenous insulin regime for labour	64	23
Blood glucose issues (mainly no targets set)	57	21
Wrong/inappropriate advice in guideline	35	13
No postnatal guideline	24	9
Out of date	19	7
No guidance on management during antenatal steroid administration	16	6
No advice on screening or management of diabetes complications	9	3
Not referenced	6	2
Recommends routine admission of baby to neonatal unit	6	2

* hospital protocols not available or data missing for 56 women.

10.6 Communication

Effective communication between health professionals, and between health professionals and women, is vital to achieving a high standard of clinical care which is responsive and puts the needs of the woman first.

10.6.1 Deficiencies in communication between health professionals

Enquiry panels assessed that there were deficiencies of communication between health professionals for 56% (222/398) of women (table 10.3). Poor communication between maternity staff and diabetes specialist teams occurred mainly during antenatal hospital admission and after delivery. Poor communication between disciplines alluded mainly to failure of the antenatal team to refer to other specialists such as renal physicians, cardiologists and ophthalmologists, with some comments made about poor transfer of information from midwifery and junior obstetric staff to more senior obstetricians during labour. Problems noted with the multidisciplinary diabetes team included a lack of a dedicated joint clinic and poor sharing of information between the obstetrician and diabetes physician.

Table 10.3

Panel comments on deficiencies of communication between health professionals caring for women with type 1 and type 2 diabetes (table contains information following categorisation of free text)

	Number of women with deficiencies in communication (N=222)	
	No. of comments	% of women
Total comments	*258*	-
Poor communication between secondary care disciplines	59	27
Poor communication between diabetes antenatal team and obstetric/midwifery staff	61	27
Problems within the multidisciplinary diabetes team	45	21
Poor communication between primary and secondary care	44	20
Poor documentation	20	9
Issue not described	20	9
Poor communication between secondary care and other health or social agencies	9	4

* 7 panel comments did not relate to communication issues

10.6.2 Deficiencies of communication between health professionals and women

Enquiry panels assessed that there were deficiencies of communication between health professionals and women for 47% (169/360) of women. The main issue seemed to be a lack of discussion between professionals and women about risks and plans for care, which occurred in nearly two thirds of the women for whom there were concerns (table 10.4).

Table 10.4

Panel comments on deficiencies of communication between health professionals and women with type 1 and type 2 diabetes (table contains information following categorisation of free text)

	Number of women with deficiencies in communication (N=169)	
	No. of comments	% of women
*Total comments**	*193*	
Suboptimal discussion about risks	77	46
Plan of care not discussed	31	18
Lack of professional interpreters for women with language difficulties	23	14
Problem within health service (poor inter-professional communication, poor follow-up, clinician's attitude etc)	19	11
Communication affected by social/lifestyle factors relating to woman	17	10
Wrong or conflicting information given	15	9
Documentation	11	7

* There were 5 comments where the issues were not described by panels

10.7 Conclusions

It is encouraging that the majority of pregnant women with pre-existing diabetes first accessed the hospital antenatal clinic within the first trimester of pregnancy and three quarters attended a combined antenatal clinic. However, just over a fifth of women in the enquiry were documented to have all members of the multidisciplinary team involved in their care, with the dietitian and midwife being the professionals least likely to be involved. While there may have been variations in interpretation of the term 'midwife with special interest in diabetes', patterns of working should be reviewed by local multidisciplinary teams to ensure that all women are receiving equivalent care and advice.

In both the obstetric and diabetes antenatal notes, there was poor documentation about what care had been given and the plans for care. Many panels had concerns that the design of the maternity hand held notes were not fit for purpose.

For nearly two thirds of women, there were concerns about local diabetes guidelines. The main issues were a lack of clarity and insufficient detail, no antenatal guidelines, inadequate intravenous insulin regimes and no guidance on blood glucose targets in labour.

There were concerns about communication between health professionals for half of women in the enquiry. A particular issue appeared to be poor lines of communication between the general maternity staff and the diabetes specialist team, and poor information sharing within the diabetes multidisciplinary team.

Documentation:

- 'No difference from normal antenatal notes so no space to record observation plans relevant to diabetes.'
- 'No diabetic entries in the obstetric notes (if she had attended another unit there would have been no record in her hand held notes).'
- 'Big gaps in documentation. Very few glucose results included in notes.'

Communication:

- 'Infrequent visits offered. Poor communication between obstetricians and physicians during pregnancy. Little or no dietitian input.'
- 'Prolonged delay after referral before being seen. Poor communication with diabetic team postnatally - did not seem to get response.'
- 'Difficulties with communication, interpreter needed, relatives used including children. Missed opportunity re advice prior to Ramadan festival.'
- 'Hypoglycaemia awareness not addressed and no apparent warning re driving.'

Guidelines:

- 'No target ranges. Sliding scale not adequate, too restrictive, would not maintain blood glucose levels appropriately.'
- 'No protocol for antenatal care or for steroid administration.'
- 'Wrong advice re Breastfeeding - protocol stated that it increased insulin requirements and risk of infection.'
- 'Protocol suggesting attendance at a combined clinic beginning only at 26/40 is considered inappropriate/poor practice.'
- 'Rigid Delivery Day. No targets for blood glucose control. Routine admission of baby to NNU.'

10.8 Recommendations

Clinical

1. Commissioners should recognise the complexity of diabetes management immediately before and during pregnancy, and ensure that the available service provision includes all members of the multidisciplinary team.
2. Patient pathways of care including preconception counselling, pregnancy care and post-pregnancy management should be incorporated into the clinical record.
3. Services should review their local guidelines. The NICE Diabetes in Pregnancy guideline, due to be published in November 2007, is anticipated to provide current evidence for best practice.

4. In order to raise awareness, it is recommended that the specialist multidisciplinary team should provide regular educational days for all primary and secondary care professionals likely to be involved in the care of women with diabetes in the local population, to cover all aspects of preconception, pregnancy and postnatal care.

Audit and research

5. Diabetes networks should carry out regular audits of preconception and pregnancy services.

References

1. *National Service Framework for Diabetes (England) Standards.* Department of Health. The Stationery Office: London: 2001.
2. *Confidential Enquiry into Maternal and Child Health. Survey of maternity services for women with type 1 and type 2 diabetes in 2002-03, England, Wales and Northern Ireland.* CEMACH: London; 2004.
3. Jardine Brown C, Dawson A, Dodds R, Gamsu H, Gillmer M, Hall M, et al. *Report of the Pregnancy and Neonatal Care Group.* Diabetic Med 1996;13:S43-S53.
4. *Clinical Negligence Scheme for Trusts Maternity Clinical Risk Management Standards.* NHS Litigation Authority. April 2006.

Commentary

John Scarpello
Deputy Medical Director, National Patient Safety Agency
Consultant Diabetes Physician, University Hospital of North Staffordshire

The CEMACH Diabetes Programme has raised important issues for those providing maternity services for women with diabetes. The CEMACH survey of diabetes maternity services showed an encouraging increase in the support available to women and most of the trusts surveyed had established combined multidisciplinary clinics. However, despite these developments, areas of unsatisfactory practice remain. All members of the multidisciplinary team were only involved in 22% of women in the enquiry and, surprisingly, dietitians were often absent. Dietetic support is important for both maternal and fetal nutrition but is also especially valuable in optimising glycaemic control, which is vital to a successful outcome.

Women with type 1 and type 2 diabetes require careful pre-pregnancy assessment with excellent glycaemic control and folic acid supplementation before conception. Once pregnancy is confirmed prompt referral is required to the multidisciplinary diabetes and obstetric team. The present enquiry has shown several areas where management is suboptimal. These include little evidence of pre-pregnancy planning and a lack of antenatal care guidelines.

Diabetes management is now more often provided by primary care rather than the secondary care specialist diabetes service. Whilst there may be advantages to this model for many people with diabetes, the management of women with diabetes of childbearing age demands agreed patient pathways and joint working between primary and secondary providers. The enquiry has found evidence of poor documentation in clinical records, and in many cases the design of the maternity notes was described as not fit for purpose. The enquiry has also highlighted deficiencies in communication between the multidisciplinary team and other disciplines, for example, general maternity staff, renal physicians, cardiologists and ophthalmologists.

Providers of diabetes maternity services should ensure that agreed standards have been documented in the patient care records, including records of diabetes complications, glycaemic control and blood pressure. Postnatal care plans should include contraceptive advice, insulin management while breastfeeding and targets for glycaemic control. Those providing diabetes maternity services will need to demonstrate that their multidisciplinary team is working to agreed patient pathways and evidence-based standards. The multi-professional team must include specialists (diabetes specialist nurses, obstetric and diabetology consultants, midwives and dietitians) trained in the management of diabetes pregnancy.

Unfortunately, the outcomes of pregnancy for women with diabetes remain poor compared to outcomes for the general maternity population. This report challenges policy makers and commissioners to improve the services provided to this high risk group of women.

11. A comparison of type 1 and type 2 diabetes

> **Learning points**
>
> - Women with type 2 diabetes in pregnancy were more likely to be obese compared to women with type 1 diabetes.
>
> - Planned pregnancy rates were similar for women with type 1 and type 2 diabetes but women with type 2 diabetes were less likely to have evidence of contraceptive use in the 12 months before pregnancy.
>
> - Women with type 2 diabetes were less likely than women with type 1 diabetes to have had a retinal assessment or test for albuminuria in the 12 months before pregnancy.
>
> - Women with type 1 diabetes in pregnancy were more likely to have retinopathy, recurrent hypoglycaemia and severe hypoglycaemic episodes than women with type 2 diabetes. Nevertheless, a fifth of women with type 2 diabetes had recurrent hypoglycaemia and 5% had new retinopathy in pregnancy.
>
> - Women with type 2 diabetes were less likely than women with type 1 diabetes to have a retinal assessment in the first trimester of pregnancy and less likely to receive postnatal contraceptive advice.

11.1 Introduction

The prevalence of type 2 diabetes is increasing[1] and the CEMACH report on 3808 pregnancies in women with pre-existing diabetes in England, Wales and Northern Ireland found that more than a quarter (27%) of women with pre-existing diabetes had type 2 diabetes.[2] Women with type 2 diabetes were a very different group to women with type 1 diabetes being more likely to be older, multiparous, from a Black, Asian and Other ethnic minority group and resident in an area of social deprivation.[2] Women with type 2 diabetes were also less likely to have had pre-pregnancy counselling, preconception folic acid and a test of glycaemic control in the 6 months before pregnancy.[2]

The enquiry module of the CEMACH Diabetes programme therefore set out to provide additional information about the differences between women with type 1 and type 2 diabetes, in terms of clinical characteristics, social and lifestyle issues, and the care provided to women.

11.2 Methodology

All women selected for the main enquiry as the control group (n=220) were included in the analyses for this chapter. In addition, 79 extra type 2 diabetic pregnancies resulting in a good outcome were also included (see Chapter 4). This gave a total of 170 women with type 1 diabetes and 127 women with type 2 diabetes, which represented 7.2% and 14.4% of all women with type 1 diabetes and type 2 diabetes respectively having a good pregnancy outcome in the full descriptive study population of 3808 pregnancies. In order to analyse a representative sample of women with type 1 and type 2 diabetes from the descriptive study, we therefore selected 7.2% of pregnancies to women with type 1 diabetes resulting in a poor pregnancy outcome and 14.4% of pregnancies to women with type 2 diabetes with a poor pregnancy outcome.

This chapter therefore relates to 181 women with type 1 diabetes (170 with good pregnancy outcome and 11 with poor pregnancy outcome) and 137 women with type 2 diabetes (127 with good pregnancy outcome and 10 with poor pregnancy outcome).

11.3 Clinical characteristics

11.3.1 Body Mass Index

Women with type 2 diabetes were more likely to have a high Body Mass Index (BMI) than women with type 1 diabetes ($\chi 2$ test for trend p<0.001, table 11.1). This was as expected, as type 2 diabetes is known to be associated with obesity.

Table 11.1

Maternal obesity in women with pre-existing diabetes

Body Mass Index (BMI)	Women with type 1 diabetes n (%) (N=181)	Women with type 2 diabetes n (%) (N=137)
18.5-24	57 (48)	12 (16)
25-29	45 (38)	17 (22)
≥ 30	18 (15)	47 (62)
Missing	61	61

11.3.2 Antenatal evidence of macrosomia and fetal growth restriction

There was no difference in the proportion of women with type 1 or type 2 diabetes with antenatal evidence of macrosomia, which was defined for the enquiry as evidence of fetal size greater than the 90th centile (p=0.99, table 11.2). This was despite the fact that a greater proportion of women with type 2 diabetes had a BMI greater than 30. However, women with type 2 diabetes were also more likely to be from an Asian ethnic minority group than women with type 1 diabetes, and their babies may not have met the enquiry definition of macrosomia (fetal size greater than the 90th centile) using standard antenatal fetal growth charts, even if it was macrosomic for an Asian population.

There was no observed difference between women with type 1 or type 2 diabetes regarding antenatal evidence of fetal growth restriction, although the absolute numbers were small (p=0.31, table 11.2).

Table 11.2

Antenatal evidence of fetal growth restriction or macrosomia in women with pre-existing diabetes

	Women with type 1 diabetes n/N (%)	Women with type 2 diabetes n/N (%)	p-value
Antenatal evidence of fetal growth restriction	11/178 (6)	12/129 (9)	0.31
Antenatal evidence of macrosomia	63/176 (36)	45/126 (36)	0.99

11.3.3 Retinopathy in pregnancy

Women with pre-existing diabetes are at risk of deterioration of existing retinopathy and development of new retinopathy during pregnancy.[3,4]

In the enquiry, retinopathy was present in more women with type 1 diabetes than in type 2 diabetes (p<0.001,table 11.3). Of the women who had retinopathy, this was a new finding for 26% of women with type 1 diabetes and also for 5 out of 9 women with type 2 diabetes (table 11.3). This highlights the importance of regular retinal assessment in pregnancy for all women with pre-existing diabetes.

Table 11.3			
Retinopathy in pregnancy in women with type 1 and type 2 diabetes			
	Women with type 1 diabetes n/N (%)	Women with type 2 diabetes n/N (%)	p-value
Retinopathy in pregnancy	50/138 (36)	9/96 (9)	P<0.001
Pre-existing – no change	25/50 (50)	3/9 (33)	-
Pre-existing and deteriorating	9/50 (18)	1/9 (11)	-
New finding	13/50 (26)	5/9 (56)	-

11.3.4 Nephropathy in pregnancy

In the enquiry, 8% (12/148) of pregnant women with type 1 diabetes and 5% (6/119) of women with type 2 diabetes had nephropathy. This was not a significant difference (p=0.32).

11.3.5 Hypoglycaemia in pregnancy

Women with diabetes are at increased risk of hypoglycaemic episodes during pregnancy due to the need to have tighter glycaemic control and also due to 'hypoglycaemia unawareness'.[5]

In the enquiry, 61% of women with type 1 diabetes had recurrent hypoglycaemic episodes during pregnancy, and nearly a fifth had a hypoglycaemic episode severe enough to require external help (Table 11.4). This reflects the difficulty in achieving optimal glycaemic control with currently available insulin therapies. Women with type 2 diabetes were less likely than women with type 1 diabetes to experience recurrent or severe hypoglycaemic episodes (p<0.001) although it is of note that 21% of women with type 2 diabetes were documented as having recurrent episodes of hypoglycaemia. The enquiry did not collect information about the proportion of women with type 2 diabetes that were on insulin during pregnancy so we are unable to report on any association between insulin use in pregnancies to women with type 2 diabetes and hypoglycaemia during pregnancy.

Table 11.4			
Hypoglycaemia during pregnancy in women with pre-existing diabetes			
	Women with type 1 diabetes n/N (%)	Women with type 2 diabetes n/N (%)	p-value
Recurrent episodes of hypoglycaemia	105/171 (61)	25/121 (21)	<0.001
One or more episode of hypoglycaemia requiring help	33/133 (25)	4/102 (4)	<0.001

11.4 Preconception behaviour

The CEMACH report on 3808 pregnancies in women with pre-existing diabetes found a poor level of pregnancy preparation, which was more marked for women with type 2 diabetes.[2] The enquiry module provided the opportunity to examine differences in other aspects of preconception behaviour.

11.4.1 Planned pregnancy and contraceptive use

Planned pregnancy rates were similar for women with type 1 diabetes (60% of 121 women) and type 2 diabetes (62% of 84 women) (p=0.73, table 11.5), compared to a planned pregnancy rate of 58% in the UK in 2001-2002.[6] However, fewer women with type 2 diabetes had evidence of contraceptive use in the 12 months prior to pregnancy (p=0.001, table 11.5). This suggests that for women with type 2 diabetes, planning a pregnancy does not necessarily equate to the use of contraception when not actively trying to conceive. This may be linked to cultural beliefs and attitudes, and health professionals need to explore these issues during annual diabetes reviews and pre-pregnancy counselling.

11.4.2 Folic acid

In the 2005 CEMACH report, 39% of all women were documented in the maternity notes or medical professional correspondence to have commenced folic acid before pregnancy, with fewer women with type 2 diabetes documented to have started folic acid in the preconception period.[2] For the enquiry module, general practitioners and the adult diabetes service were asked to provide information on folic acid use before pregnancy. A higher rate of preconception folic acid use than for the full cohort was reported (49% of women with type 1 diabetes and 45% of women with type 2 diabetes), and there was no observed difference between folic acid use in the two groups of women (p=0.60, Table 11.5).

The difference in findings between the descriptive study and the enquiry may be due to the fact that the information on folic acid in the descriptive study was dependent on documentation in the maternity notes, whereas in the enquiry, adult diabetes services and general practitioners were approached for information. It is also possible that health professionals were less likely to document folic acid use in the maternity notes or general medical records for women with type 2 diabetes than for women with type 1 diabetes, perhaps due to issues such as language difficulties.

Table 11.5			
Preconception behaviour in women with pre-existing diabetes			
	Women with type 1 diabetes n/N (%)	Women with type 2 diabetes n/N (%)	p-value
Planned pregnancy	72/121 (60)	52/84 (62)	0.73
Evidence of contraceptive use in the 12 months prior to pregnancy	61/104 (59)	21/65 (32)	0.001
Evidence of preconception folic acid	54/110 (49)	32/71 (45)	0.60
Smoking	41/150 (27)	22/108 (20)	0.20
Assessment of suboptimal approach of the woman to managing her diabetes before pregnancy	83/135 (61)	51/88 (60)	0.60
Assessment of suboptimal approach of the woman to managing her diabetes during pregnancy	50/171 (29)	36/124 (29)	0.97

11.5 Preconception care in the 12 months prior to pregnancy

There were no differences between women with type 1 and type 2 diabetes in terms of the contraceptive advice, specific diabetes advice and information about pregnancy risks and surveillance provided by clinicians before pregnancy (table 11.6) However, women with type 2 diabetes were less likely to have a retinal examination and assessment of albuminuria than women with type 1 diabetes in the 12 months before pregnancy (p=0.004, p=0.04 respectively, table 11.6).

Table 11.6
Differences in preconception care between women with type 1 and type 2 diabetes

	Women with type 1 diabetes n/N (%)	Women with type 2 diabetes n/N (%)	p-value
No contraceptive advice given	18/76 (24)	18/44 (41)	0.05
No recorded discussion of the following specific diabetes issues:			
Alcohol intake	16/57 (28)	8/30 (27)	0.09
Diet	10/82 (12)	5/56 (9)	0.55
Poor glycaemic control	12/102 (12)	4/60 (7)	0.29
Retinopathy	17/80 (21)	11/37 (30)	0.31
Nephropathy	21/64 (33)	14/29 (48)	0.15
Hypertension	19/64 (30)	11/32 (34)	0.64
No recorded discussion of the following pregnancy issues:			
Increased diabetes surveillance	7/109 (6)	4/57 (7)	0.88
Increased pregnancy surveillance	8/109 (7)	4/56 (7)	0.96
Increased risk of induction	13/95 (14)	8/40 (20)	0.36
Possible caesarean section	11/93 (12)	6/47 (13)	0.87
Fetal risks in diabetic pregnancy	7/97 (7)	4/48 (8)	0.81
No dietetic review	87/110 (79)	19/77 (25)	0.19
No assessment of the following diabetes complications in the 12 months prior to pregnancy:			
Baseline retinal examination	12/122 (10)	17/66 (26)	0.004
Baseline test of renal function	10/115 (9)	21/175 (12)	0.06
Assessment of albuminuria	20/92 (22)	21/56 (38)	0.04
Assessment of suboptimal preconception care (apart from glycaemic control)	72/116 (62)	53/72 (74)	0.1

11.6 Glycaemic control

There was no difference in the proportion of women with type 1 or type 2 diabetes having a test of glycaemic control in the 12 months before pregnancy (table 11.7). This was different to the findings of the descriptive study, where women with type 2 diabetes were less likely than women with type 1 diabetes to have documented evidence of a pre-pregnancy test of glycaemic control.[2] This may be because the enquiry related to a 12 month prior to pregnancy rather than 6 months as for the descriptive study. Also, in the descriptive study, information was dependent on documentation in the maternity notes whereas in the enquiry, the adult diabetes service and general practitioner were also approached for information, and this may have resulted in increased ascertainment.

Women with type 1 diabetes were more likely than women with type 2 diabetes to have suboptimal preconception glycaemic control as assessed by enquiry panels (table 11.7). This was similar to the descriptive study, where only 24% of 1081 women with type 1 diabetes had a median HbA1c less than 7% prior to pregnancy compared to 41% of 303 women with type 2 diabetes.[2]

Fewer women with type 2 diabetes received intravenous insulin and dextrose during delivery (table 11.7). This finding may partly reflect the fact that a proportion of women with type 2 diabetes do not require insulin during pregnancy. Also, women with type 2 diabetes were more likely to be multiparous[2], and there may have been no opportunity in labour to commence intravenous insulin and dextrose.

Table 11.7

Differences in factors related to glycaemic control between women with type 1 and type 2 diabetes

	Women with type 1 diabetes n/N (%)	Women with type 2 diabetes n/N (%)	p-value
No test of glycaemic control in the 12 months prior to pregnancy	20/120 (17)	14/73 (19)	0.66
No evidence of local targets set for glycaemic control	24/73 (33)	11/34 (32)	0.96
Assessment of suboptimal preconception glycaemic control	105/140 (75)	58/97 (60)	0.013
Assessment of suboptimal 1st trimester glycaemic control	104/160 (65)	66/122 (54)	0.064
Assessment of suboptimal glycaemic control after 1st trimester	71/174 (41)	46/130 (35)	0.34
Assessment of suboptimal blood glucose control during labour and delivery	78/165 (47)	49/120 (41)	0.28
No intravenous insulin and dextrose during labour and/or delivery	18/180 (10)	38/133 (29)	<0.001

11.7 Clinical care during pregnancy

It is encouraging that there did not appear to be any differences in maternity care during the antenatal period between women with type 1 and type 2 diabetes (table 11.8) However, fewer women with type 2 diabetes had a retinal assessment in the first trimester of pregnancy (table 11.9). This is of concern when it is considered that 5 women with type 2 diabetes had new retinopathy diagnosed during pregnancy (table 11.3).

Table 11.8

Differences in maternity care during the antenatal period between women with type 1 and type 2 diabetes

	Women with type 1 diabetes n/N (%)	Women with type 2 diabetes n/N (%)	p-value
Assessment of suboptimal fetal monitoring (with antenatal evidence of growth restricted baby)	2/11 (18)	1/11 (9)	0.53
Assessment of suboptimal fetal monitoring (with antenatal evidence of big baby > 90th centile)	19/32 (59)	16/45 (36)	0.68
No discussion of mode and timing of delivery	5/164 (3)	4/122 (3)	0.91
No administration of corticosteroids	9/28 (32)	8/24 (33)	0.93
Assessment of suboptimal maternity care during the antenatal period	76/177 (43)	70/131 (53)	0.07
Assessment of suboptimal maternity care during labour and delivery	59/178 (33)	56/131 (43)	0.08

Table 11.9

Differences in diabetes care (excluding glycaemic control) during pregnancy between women with type 1 and type 2 diabetes

	Women with type 1 diabetes n/N (%)	Women with type 2 diabetes n/N (%)	p-value
No retinal assessment	33/148 (22)	42/117 (36)	0.02
No referral to ophthalmologist (if retinopathy present)	20/43 (47)	5/9 (56)	0.62
No monitoring for nephropathy	24/169 (14)	21/128 (16)	0.6
No test of renal function (if nephropathy present)	3/12 (25)	3/6 (50)	0.29
Assessment of suboptimal diabetes care during pregnancy	96/169 (57)	49/120 (41)	0.28

11.8 Postnatal care

Women with type 2 diabetes were less likely to receive postnatal contraceptive advice than women with type 1 diabetes (table 11.10). This may have been due partly to language difficulties and also perceived differences in cultural attitudes to contraception. All women with pre-existing diabetes should receive advice about contraception soon after delivery in order to prevent future unplanned pregnancies, and it should be agreed locally as to which professionals are best placed to provide this advice in the puerperium.

Table 11.10

Differences in postnatal care between women with type 1 and type 2 diabetes

	Women with type 1 diabetes n/N (%)	Women with type 2 diabetes n/N (%)	p-value
No postnatal contraceptive advice	21/137 (15)	31/105 (30)	0.008
No written plan for post-delivery diabetes management	20/156 (13)	15/115 (13)	0.95
Assessment of suboptimal postnatal diabetes care	93/177 (53)	59/127 (46)	0.3

11.9 Conclusions

The comparison of women with type 1 and type 2 diabetes has shown some differences in clinical characteristics (Body Mass Index, retinopathy and frequency and severity of hypoglycaemia in pregnancy) which are to be expected from the difference in disease profiles between the two groups of women.

It is concerning that women with type 2 diabetes were less likely than women with type 1 diabetes to have a retinal assessment in the first trimester (or at booking if later), especially since retinopathy was a new finding in five out of the nine women with type 2 diabetes who had retinopathy in pregnancy. This may reflect a perception by health professionals that type 2 diabetes is less likely to cause complications than type 1 diabetes, and highlights the importance of early and regular retinal assessment for all women with pre-existing diabetes.

Before pregnancy, women with type 2 diabetes were less likely than women with type 1 diabetes to have a retinal assessment or test for albuminuria in the 12 months before pregnancy. Women with type 2 diabetes are more likely to be managed in primary care, and this finding may therefore reflect a lack of awareness by primary care professionals of the importance of screening for diabetes complications in women with type 2 diabetes. There may also be difficulties in accessing investigations such as retinal photographs that are usually provided in the secondary care setting.

Women with type 2 diabetes were less likely to receive postnatal contraceptive advice. It is recognised that health professionals may find it difficult to provide contraceptive advice to women from different cultural backgrounds due to language difficulties and perceived cultural sensitivities. However, this is a vital aspect of post-delivery counselling, and every effort should be made by health professionals to help women with diabetes, including those with type 2 diabetes, to prepare adequately for future pregnancies.

11.10 Recommendations

Clinical

1. During pregnancy, retinal and renal screening schedules should be provided for both women with type 1 and women with type 2 diabetes.
2. Advice about hypoglycaemia during pregnancy, including prevention and management strategies, should be provided to both women with type 1 diabetes and women with type 2 diabetes.

Audit and research

3. Diabetes networks should audit standards of preconception and pregnancy care for both women with type 1 and women with type 2 diabetes.

References

1. Lusignan S, Sismanidis C, Carey IM, DeWilde S, Richards N, Cook DG. *Trends in the prevalence and management of diagnosed type 2 diabetes 1994-2001 in England and Wales.* BMC Family Practice 6(1), 2 Mar 2005: 13.
2. *Confidential Enquiry into Maternal and Child Health. Pregnancy in women with type 1 and type 2 diabetes in 2002-03, England, Wales and Northern Ireland.* CEMACH: London; 2005.
3. Sheth BP. *Does pregnancy accelerate the rate of progression of diabetic retinopathy?* Current Diabetes Reports 2(4), Aug 2002: 327-30.
4. Temple RC, Aldridge VA, Sampson MJ, Greenwood RH, Heyburn PJ, Glenn A. *Impact of pregnancy on the progression of diabetic retinopathy in Type 1 diabetes. Diabetic Medicine.* Jul 2001: 18(7): 573-7.
5. ter Braak EW, Evers IM, Erkelens DW, Visser GH.*Maternal hypoglycaemia during pregnancy in type 1 diabetes: maternal and fetal consequences.* Diabetes Metab Res Rev 2002; 18:96-105.
6. Dex S, Heather J (eds). *Millennium Cohort Study First Survey: a user's guide to initial findings.* Centre for Longitudinal Studies: London; 2004.

Commentary

Robert Fraser
Chair, NICE Diabetes in Pregnancy Guideline Development Group
Consultant Obstetrician, Royal Hallamshire Hospital, Sheffield

The proportionate distribution of type 1 and type 2 diabetes in women with diabetes during pregnancy is changing, with an increasing number of pregnancies in women with type 2 diabetes being seen. This is due to a rapid increase in the prevalence of obesity in all ethnic groups in the population, obesity occurring in younger people, and a rise in age specific maximum fertility. The importance of mature onset diabetes of youth (MODY) is also becoming recognised amongst younger women with type 2 diabetes and this group bring their own particular problems to pregnancy management which deserve separate and detailed management guidelines.

Type 1 and type 2 diabetes have traditionally been managed differently. As the prevalence of type 2 diabetes in pregnancy increases, it is appropriate to review how we manage women of childbearing age with known type 2 diabetes. Also, women with gestational diabetes (GDM) are at increased risk of type 2 diabetes after pregnancy, and in some populations up to 20% of women diagnosed to have gestational diabetes actually have previously undiagnosed type 2 diabetes. This brings them into a high risk group for future pregnancies, and although this report did not address gestational diabetes, these women may also benefit from properly structured management strategies including pre-pregnancy care.

Although retinopathy is much less common in women with type 2 diabetes it is present in a significant minority and they are presumably equally vulnerable to deterioration of retinopathy during pregnancy. They therefore need to be enrolled in a suitable annual review outside pregnancy, either in primary or secondary care. They are likely to benefit as much as women with type 1 diabetes from digital retinal photography.

In the CEMACH enquiry, unplanned pregnancy and preconception folic acid use was equivalent in women with type 1 and type 2 diabetes, and women with type 2 diabetes appeared less likely to use contraception. It is important that both groups of women should have messages reinforced about pregnancy preparation. During pregnancy, it is clear that women with type 2 diabetes should have the same standard of maternal and fetal surveillance as women with type 1 diabetes. However, women with type 2 diabetes have a relative rarity of severe hypoglycaemia requiring third party assistance.

During labour, fewer women with type 2 diabetes receive intravenous insulin and dextrose; this is perhaps a reflection of reasonable clinical practice in that these women may very well have shorter labours and are certainly at less risk of serious metabolic disturbance during labour.

The finding that women with type 2 diabetes are less likely to receive postnatal contraceptive advice is of concern, and the importance of providing contraceptive advice to this particular group of women must be emphasised through adult diabetes services and general practitioners. It may also be worthwhile to extend education about the pregnancy risks for women with type 2 diabetes to other primary care health professionals such as Family Planning practitioners and nurses.

12. Neonatal care of term babies

Learning points

- One third of admissions to a neonatal unit occurred because of a unit policy of routinely admitting well babies of mothers with diabetes. Enquiry panels assessed that over half of all neonatal admissions were avoidable.

- Several barriers to breastfeeding were reported:
  - Lack of early close maternal contact and early feeding on the labour ward
  - High rate of infant formula given as first feed
  - Infant formula given to all babies admitted to a neonatal unit, even when the maternal intention was to breastfeed
  - Infant formula feeding on the postnatal ward often explained by maternal choice.

- Blood glucose testing often took place too early with inappropriate methods of testing used; documentation of blood glucose tests was poor.

- Two thirds of babies were assessed to have suboptimal neonatal care on the delivery suite; this frequently affected subsequent care.

- A quarter of medical records did not have a written management plan.

12.1 Introduction

In 2002, 30% of hospitals in England, Wales and Northern Ireland reported that they routinely admitted babies of women with diabetes to a neonatal unit.[1] In addition, the CEMACH descriptive study of 3808 pregnancies to women with type 1 and type 2 diabetes found substandard neonatal management of hypoglycaemia and early feeding; a lower intention to breastfeed in mothers with diabetes at birth than in the general population; and a higher number than expected admissions of term babies to a neonatal unit.[2] It was therefore decided to carry out an additional enquiry into the neonatal care of term babies of women with diabetes in the CEMACH Diabetes Programme. The key findings are summarised in this chapter.

12.2 Methodology

12.2.1 Composition and location of enquiry panels

Enquiry panel meetings were held in five CEMACH regions (East of England, London, North East, North West and South West) between January and April 2006. Each panel consisted of two representatives from each of the following disciplines:

- Neonatologists
- Neonatal nurses
- Midwives.

Panels were chaired by the panel chairs appointed for the Diabetes Enquiry or by the CEMACH regional manager of that region. Six cases were reviewed at each meeting. Cases reviewed were selected from a national pool excluding the region of the assessing panel, to ensure an independent assessment of the care provided. Each panel was provided with neonatal records and charts pertaining to the first three days after delivery, discharge summaries, the postnatal maternity notes, any relevant correspondence and hospital protocols.

12.2.2 Enquiry pro forma

Clinical guidance for the neonatal enquiry was provided by a steering group of clinicians with specific experience in neonatal care for babies of women with diabetes (Appendix F). A structured enquiry pro forma (accessible at www.cemach.org.uk) was developed in consultation with members of the steering group. This pro forma was designed to assess neonatal care provided on the labour ward, the postnatal ward or on the neonatal unit.

12.2.3 Standards of care

Care was assessed against standards relating to the location of care, blood glucose monitoring, temperature management and feeding. The clinical standards for this enquiry were those used in the CEMACH Diabetes Programme (accessible at www.cemach.org.uk), with some additional standards from the Baby Friendly Initiative [3]

12.2.4 Enquiry sample

In the neonatal enquiry, pregnancies were randomly sampled from the diabetes cohort database of 3808 pregnancies after excluding deaths, fetal congenital anomalies, multiple births and gestation at delivery less than 37+0 weeks. The case definition for the neonatal enquiry was therefore all term pregnancies in women with diabetes resulting in a normally formed baby surviving to 28 days after delivery. One hundred and thirty two babies met this case definition. Neonatal medical records were not available for 13 babies, leaving 119 babies for enquiry. These babies were then divided into two groups for further comparative analysis:

- babies who were initially admitted with their mother to the postnatal ward or to a transitional care unit[a], or who stayed with their mother on the labour ward or a maternal high dependency unit
- babies who were initially admitted to a neonatal unit for special care.[b]

[a] defined as units where, if baby needs non intensive treatment and monitoring, mothers and babies can be cared for together under supervision of neonatal staff.

[b] Care provided for all babies not receiving intensive or high dependency care but whose carers could not reasonably be expected to look after them in hospital or at home (British Association of Perinatal Medicine 2001).

12.3 The babies in the neonatal enquiry

In the 119 babies selected for neonatal enquiry, two sets of medical records were not available and five babies had no documented location of care. Amongst the remaining 112 babies with data available on their care in the first three days of life, 70 babies were nursed initially with their mothers (61 on the postnatal ward, five in a transitional care unit and four on the labour ward or maternal high dependency unit). By day three, nearly half of these 70 babies had been discharged from hospital. Six babies, who were initially nursed with their mother, were later admitted to a neonatal unit.

Forty two babies were admitted directly to a neonatal unit after delivery. By day three, one third of these 42 babies were still on the unit while two thirds had returned to be with their mothers on the postnatal ward. Two babies were later readmitted to the neonatal unit.

12.4 Avoidable admissions

Current national guidance is that babies of women with diabetes should be admitted to a neonatal unit only if there is a specific medical indication.[5-7] As already mentioned, in 2002, a third of units routinely admitted babies of women with diabetes to the neonatal unit.[1] The CEMACH descriptive study also found that 30% of term babies were admitted to a neonatal unit[2], a threefold increase over the neonatal admission rate in the general maternity population in the UK.[4] This is concerning, as separation of mother and baby after birth may affect a number of important processes such as early establishment of breastfeeding, temperature control and emotional bonding.

12.4.1 Enquiry findings

The three main indications for admission to a neonatal unit were a hospital policy of routine admission of healthy babies of mothers with diabetes; non-symptomatic hypoglycaemia in a healthy baby; and a clinical need for admission such as poor feeding and respiratory problems.

Table 12.1	
Reasons for admission of babies of mothers with diabetes to a neonatal unit	
	Babies admitted to a neonatal unit n (%) (N=42)
Hospital policy (infant of mother with diabetes)	12 (29)
Non symptomatic hypoglycaemia in a well baby	11 (26)
Baby clinically needing admission:	18 (43)
Hypothermia (with hypoglycaemia)	6
Poor feeding (with hypoglycaemia)	3
Macrosomia (otherwise well baby)	3
Respiratory difficulties	5
Other medical condition (cardiac)	1
Not known	1 (0)

In 57% (24/42) of cases, a junior doctor (senior house officer in paediatrics) made the decision to admit a baby to the neonatal unit. Enquiry panels assessed that 57% (24/42) of admissions could have been avoided, with subsequent care being adversely affected for 63% (15/24) of the babies. The main area of care affected by an avoidable admission was feeding, for 50% (12/24) of the babies.

12.4.2 Panel comments on avoidable admissions

Enquiry panels made 24 comments for 24 babies about avoidable admissions. The most frequent comment, for 63% (15/24) of babies, was that there was no valid medical reason to admit to the neonatal unit (table 12.2).

Table 12.2

Panel comments on avoidable admissions to a neonatal unit (table contains information following categorisation of free text)

	No. of comments	% of avoidable admissions (N=24)
Total comments	24	
No medical reason for admission	15	63
Poor management of temperature	5	21
Delay in initiating feeding	2	8
Poor maternal blood glucose management during labour/at delivery	1	4
Blood glucose tested too soon after delivery	1	4

12.5 Barriers to breastfeeding

Several studies have shown that postnatal care programmes such as the Baby Friendly initiative that help promote undisturbed mother-infant contact improve breastfeeding success.[3,8,9] These initiatives are likely to be of benefit to mothers with diabetes and their babies, who may be more vulnerable to the negative psychological impact of a high-risk medical condition in pregnancy.[10] There is evidence that babies whose mothers keep them in closer skin contact are warm, calm and reassured.[11,12] Systematic reviews of early skin contact between mothers and babies also show benefits in relation to breastfeeding and infant crying.[13]

National guidance for women with diabetes recommends breastfeeding as early as possible after delivery,[6,7] as these babies may be at risk of hypoglycaemia.[5,14] In addition, infant formula supplementation may suppress the process of normal metabolic adaptation. Breast milk is thought to promote ketogenesis[15] and should therefore be the first choice for babies of women with diabetes, as they are at risk of hypoketonaemic hypoglycaemia. However, the previous CEMACH descriptive study found that the intention to breastfeed rate in women with diabetes was lower than the initial breastfeeding rate in the general population.[2,16]

12.5.1 Enquiry findings

Early feeding and skin-to-skin contact on the labour ward

Opportunity for early skin-to-skin contact after birth (within 30 minutes of delivery, or as soon as the mother was able to respond following caesarean section) was documented to be achieved for 29% (30/102) of babies. In eight instances, skin-to-skin contact was considered not practicable because of the clinical condition of mother and/or the baby.

Seventy seven percent (75/97) of babies received their first feed while on the labour ward. Ninety five percent of babies remaining with their mothers received their first feed on the labour ward compared to 50% of babies admitted to a neonatal unit (p<0.001). It is possible that the clinical condition of a proportion of babies admitted to the neonatal unit did not allow feeding and in particular breastfeeding; however, these findings imply that at least half of the babies admitted to a neonatal unit were well enough to breastfeed.

Breastfeeding support on the labour ward

Twenty six percent (29/112) of mothers were documented to have received help with breastfeeding within the first hour after birth (34% of mothers whose babies remained with them and 12% of mothers whose babies were admitted to a neonatal unit, p=0.07). It is of concern that a third of mothers in both groups had no documented breastfeeding support despite breastfeeding being their intended method of feeding (table12.3).

Table 12.3 Documented evidence of breastfeeding support on the labour ward for women with type 1 and type 2 diabetes			
	Babies in neonatal enquiry		
Breastfeeding support	**Remaining with mother n(%) (N=70)**	**Admitted to NNU n(%) (N=42)**	**Total n(%)* (N=112)**
Yes	24 (37)	5 (13)	29 (28)
No	23 (35)	14 (35)	36 (35)
Assessed as not practicable	1 (2)	9 (23)	10 (9)
Not applicable[†]	17 (26)	12 (30)	29 (28)
Missing	5	2	7

* Percentages are calculated from all babies in relevant category excluding those where data was missing.

[†] Breastfeeding was not mother's intended method of feeding.

Breastfeeding support in the neonatal unit

Only 31% (13/42) of mothers whose babies were admitted to the neonatal unit had documented evidence in the medical records that they had been shown how to breastfeed and maintain lactation (e.g. express breast milk) when separated from their babies. Nineteen percent (8/42) of mothers did not wish to breastfeed.

Infant formula given as first feed

Infant formula was the most frequently recorded milk given at first feed (for 63%, 67/106 of babies in the enquiry) (table 12.4). Twenty nine percent of the 31 formula-fed babies admitted to a neonatal unit were fed either by a cup or by tube, but a bottle was used to give the first feed for all 36 formula-fed babies who remained with their mothers. Breast milk was the first feed for 40% of 106 babies (50%, 34/68 of babies who remained with their mothers and 21%, 8/38 of babies admitted to a neonatal unit, p=0.001).

The most frequent reason documented for infant formula being given at any feed to babies remaining with their mothers, was maternal choice, for 46% (32/70) of babies.

Table 12.4

Type of milk at first feed for babies of women with type 1 and type 2 diabetes

	Babies remaining with mother n(%) (N=70*)	Babies admitted to NNU n(%) (N=42*)	Total n(%) (N=112)
Maternal breast milk	34 (50)	8 (21)	42 (40)
Donor breast milk	2 (3)	0 (0)	2 (2)
Infant formula	36 (53)	31 (82)	67 (83)
Type of milk at first feed not recorded	2	4	6

* some babies had more than one option for first feed ticked.

Intention to breastfeed

The first feed given was not the mothers' intended type of feed for 28% (27/96) of babies (16% of babies who remained with their mothers and 50% of those admitted to a neonatal unit, p<0.001)). This information was not available for 14% of babies (8 babies in each group).

Infant formula given to all babies admitted to a neonatal unit, even when maternal intention to breastfeed

The type of milk given on the neonatal unit was documented for 41/42 babies (table 12.5). Twenty eight of the 41 babies received more than one type of milk. Infant formula was the most frequently recorded first feed, being given to all the 41 babies for whom information was available.

Twenty five out of 41 babies had breast milk, always by breastfeeding.

Table 12.5

Type of milk given to babies of women with type 1 and type 2 diabetes on the neonatal unit

Type of milk*	Received only one type of milk	Received more than one type of milk	Total no. of babies (N=41)
Breast milk	0	25	25
Donor milk	0	1	1
Infant formula	13	28	41

* Babies could be fed by multiple methods but same type of milk e.g. infant formula from cup and tube.

12.5.2 Panel assessment of feeding in the neonatal unit

Panels assessed that the type of feed the baby received was appropriate in 62% (26/42) of cases.

12.5.3 Panel assessment of the impact of management in the neonatal care unit on feeding

Panels considered that management of the baby, over and above the fact of being on the neonatal unit for special care, was likely to have had a negative impact on the establishment of feeding for 38% (15/40) of all babies (46%, 11/24 when there was a maternal intention to breastfeed and 25%, 4/16 when an alternative method of feeding was intended (p=0.18) (table 12.6).

Table 12.6			
Panel assessment of the impact of management of the baby on establishment of feeding for babies of women with type 1 and type 2 diabetes on the neonatal unit			
	Maternal intention to breastfeed		
Effect of management of the baby	Yes n(%) (N=25)	No n(%) (N=17)	Total n(%)* (N=42)
Had an impact on establishment of feeding	11 (46)	4 (25)	15 (38)
Did not have an impact on establishment of feeeing	12 (50)	10 (63)	22 (55)
Not enough information	1 (4)	2 (13)	3 (8)
Missing	*1*	*1*	*2*

* Percentages are calculated from all babies in relevant category excluding those babies where data was missing.

12.6 Blood glucose management

The standard agreed for the CEMACH Diabetes Programme (standards accessible at www.cemach.org.uk) stated that babies of mothers with diabetes should have a test of blood glucose concentration by 4-6 hours of age, before a feed.[2] The previous descriptive study suggested that blood glucose testing was often performed too soon, coinciding with the physiological fall in blood glucose after birth and potentially leading to unnecessary admissions to the neonatal unit.[2]

The descriptive study also found that neonatal blood glucose testing was mainly carried out using a reagent strip technique.[2] Reagent strip testing is unreliable[17] and when considering the diagnosis of hypoglycaemia, at least one laboratory value should be obtained.[18] The suitability of using a portable glucose photometer such as the HaemoCue to diagnose neonatal hypoglycaemia is not universally accepted.[17, 19-21] Currently, national guidelines recommend that the diagnosis of neonatal hypoglycaemia in babies at increased risk should be made using ward-based glucose electrode or laboratory methods and not by reagent strip.[2,6]

12.6.1 Enquiry findings

12.6.1.1 Timing of first blood glucose testing

Babies had their first blood glucose test mainly during the first two hours of life (table 12.7). The first test was performed at a median of 1.15 hours in babies admitted to a neonatal unit and at a median of

2.1 hours in babies remaining with their mothers. The wide range in age of the baby at first blood glucose test shows that some tests were carried out almost immediately after birth. Median first blood glucose values were identical in both groups. Panels were asked if there were abnormal clinical signs attributable to hypoglycaemia at the time of the first blood glucose measurement: two babies were described as jittery with no other symptoms.

Table 12.7
Timing and result of first blood glucose measurement in term babies of women with type 1 and type 2 diabetes

	Babies remaining with mother (N=70)		Babies admitted to NNU (N=42)		p-value
Time of first blood glucose measurement (hours) (median [IQR] (range)	2.1 [0.97-4.33] (0.05 - 9.63)	N=58	1.15 [0.38-1.97] (0 - 7.6)	n=34	0.08
First blood glucose value (mmol/L) (median [IQR] (range)	2.8 [2.3-3.7] (0.8 - 9.0)	N=68	2.5 [2.0-3.3] (0.8 - 5.7)	n=39	0.42

12.6.1.2 Methods of blood glucose testing

Reagent strip testing was the main method documented. In many cases, there was no documentation of the method used (table 12.8). It was also noted that the abbreviation "BM" was often used inappropriately to denote blood glucose.

Table 12.8
Method used for first blood glucose measurement in babies of women with type 1 and type 2 diabetes

Method used	Babies in neonatal enquiry (N=112)
HaemoCue	10
Reagent strip	53
Dextrostix	0
"BM"	53
Glucose electrode method	6
Yellow springs	0
Blood gas analyser	4
Other glucose electrode method	2
Other	1
Not documented	42

Sixty eight percent of blood glucose measurement tests were done pre-feed and 26% post-feed (table 12.9). These proportions were similar for babies admitted to a neonatal unit and babies remaining with their mothers.

Table 12.9

Timing of first blood glucose measurement in relation to feed in babies of mothers with type 1 and type 2 diabetes

Timing of first blood glucose measurement	Babies remaining with mother n(%) (N=70)	Babies admitted to NNU n(%) (N=42)	Total (N=112)
Pre-feed	43 (64)	28 (74)	71 (68)
Post-feed	18 (27)	9 (24)	27 (26)
Random	6 (9)	1 (3)	7 (7)
Missing	*3*	*4*	*7*

12.6.2 Panel assessment of documentation of blood glucose management

Panels assessed that documentation of blood glucose measurements was more frequently suboptimal on the postnatal ward (81%, 57/70 of babies) than on the neonatal unit (48%, 20/42 of babies, p<0.001). Panels made 99 comments for 77 babies with suboptimal documentation of blood glucose measurements (table 12.10). The two main issues identified by panels were a lack of documentation of the methods used and no written plan for blood glucose management.

Table 12.10

Panel comments on suboptimal documentation relating to blood glucose measurements (table contains information following categorisation of free text)

	Babies with suboptimal documentation of blood glucose measurements (N=77)	
	No. of comments	% of babies
Total comments	**99**	
No documentation of methods used	30	39
No written blood glucose management plan	22	29
Pre and post-feed not specified	10	13
"BM" stated as the method of testing	10	13
Confusion due to baby's and mother's blood glucose recorded in the same notes	11	14
Poor design of notes	6	8
Timing of blood glucose testing or feeding not recorded	5	7
Notes/charts not available	3	4
Other	2	3

12.7 Panel assessment of care of babies on the labour ward

Enquiry panels assessed that care on the labour ward was suboptimal for 55% (62/112) of babies (53%, 37/70 of babies remaining with their mothers and 71%, 25/42 of those admitted to a neonatal unit, no significant difference).

12.7.1 Panel comments on suboptimal care of babies on the labour ward

Panels made 95 comments for the 62 babies whose care on the labour ward was suboptimal (table 12.11). The most frequently recorded issues were: a) inappropriate timing of blood glucose testing b) no close early contact between mother and baby/ missed breastfeeding opportunities c) allowing the baby to get cold and d) no plan of care.

Table 12.11 Panel comments on suboptimal care on the labour ward (table contains information following categorisation of free text)	Babies with suboptimal care on labour ward (N=62)	
	No. of comments	% of babies
Total comments	95	
Blood glucose	22	36
Done too soon	7	
Delayed	5	
No monitoring	2	
Substandard management	7	
No documentation	1	
Feeding	23	37
Delayed	7	
No skin-to-skin contact/breastfeeding opportunity	12	
Breastfeeding impaired/overturned	2	
Other management	1	
No documentation	1	
Temperature	29	47
Allowed to get cold	12	
No monitoring	9	
Not documented	8	
Overall management	16	26
No clinical assessment	2	
No plan of care	12	
No guidelines/protocol	2	
Other	5	8

12.8 Written management plans

It is important to have a clear written management plan at birth for babies of women with diabetes, to help staff on the neonatal unit and midwives on the postnatal ward to direct their neonatal care appropriately.

12.8.1 Enquiry findings

There was evidence of a clear written care plan for 73% (51/70) of babies who remained with their mothers and 57% (24/42) of babies admitted to a neonatal unit (table 12.12). The plan referred to a hospital protocol in a third or less of the cases, and included advice about blood glucose monitoring and feeding more consistently than for other areas of care. A temperature management plan was present in less than half of babies, and the recommended location of care was documented for a third of babies remaining with their mothers and two thirds of babies admitted to a neonatal unit. The care plan was written by the paediatric Senior House Officer for 57% (42/74) of babies and by the midwife for 15% (11/74) of babies. In 22% of cases, there was insufficient information in the notes to determine who had written the care plan.

The care plan was not fully followed for 35% (18/51) of babies remaining with their mother; aspects of the care plan not followed included blood glucose management, feeding and temperature control.

Table 12.12			
Written care plan for babies of women with type 1 and type 2 diabetes			
	Babies remaining with mother n(%)* (N=70)	Babies admitted to NNU n(%)* (N=42)	p-value
Evidence of a written plan	51 (73)	24 (57)	0.12
Plan refers to hospital protocol	17 (33)	5 (21)	0.27
Location of care	18 (35)	16 (67)	0.01
Blood glucose monitoring	47 (92)	19 (79)	0.16
Temperature management	24 (47)	7 (29)	0.14
Feeding	43 (84)	16 (67)	0.12

* Percentages are calculated for each aspect of the care plan after excluding missing data.

12.9 Conclusions

The overall findings of this enquiry into the neonatal care of term babies born to mothers with diabetes suggested that:

- There were many concerns about clinical care and documentation, especially on the labour ward:
  - Avoidable admissions had an adverse effect on the establishment of breastfeeding
  - Initial support for early mother-baby contact and breastfeeding was inconsistent
  - Timing and method of blood glucose monitoring was inconsistent.
- There was little evidence of senior paediatric staff involvement in the management of this group of babies.
- Many healthy babies of mothers with diabetes were separated from their parents without a good medical reason. The design of most maternity units, where neonatal expertise is predominantly concentrated in the neonatal unit, may partly explain why trusts are reluctant to provide care for these higher risk babies on a postnatal ward with their mothers. Bringing neonatal expertise close to the mothers as occurs in transitional care wards, may be the solution.

The concerns described here probably extend beyond the specific group of babies of mothers with diabetes. They open a national debate on whether basic neonatal care can be delivered closer to the mother in maternity units in England, Wales and Northern Ireland.

Some quotes from the panel discussions

- 'Should not have got cold, should not have gone to the neonatal unit, could have ended up breastfeeding.'
- 'This was a routine admission to the neonatal unit. Breastfeeding was not initiated and unnecessary procedures were done.'
- 'Blood glucose taken too early. This had an effect on care and the establishment of breastfeeding.'
- 'If the blood glucose had not been done so soon, mother and baby may not have needed to be separated.'
- 'Mother wanted to breastfeed, but paediatric SHO overrode this and made the feed to be infant formula.'
- 'No management plan of care when baby transferred to postnatal ward and baby was left for eight hours without a feed and not enough true blood glucose results.'

12.10 Recommendations

1. All units delivering women with diabetes should have a written policy for the management of the baby. The policy should assume that babies will remain with their mothers in the absence of complications.
2. Mothers with diabetes should be informed antenatally of the beneficial effects of breastfeeding on metabolic control for both themselves and their babies.
3. Mothers with diabetes should be offered an opportunity for skin-to-skin contact with their babies immediately after delivery. Breastfeeding within one hour of birth should be encouraged.
4. Blood glucose testing performed too early should be avoided in well babies without signs of hypoglycaemia. Testing should be performed before a feed using a reliable method (ward-based glucose electrode or laboratory analysis). For all blood glucose tests, the time it is performed, method used, result, and action taken should be clearly documented in the notes. Further research is needed to define the optimal timing of first blood glucose test in babies of diabetic mothers.
5. Junior paediatric staff should be trained in the management of babies of mothers with diabetes. This should include appreciation of the importance of supporting early breastfeeding, avoidance of early blood glucose testing in the well baby, and formulation of a written plan agreed with the mother.
6. Midwives should recognise the importance of supporting early breastfeeding for women with diabetes, and the need to document this aspect of care.

References

1. *Confidential Enquiry into Maternal and Child Health. Maternity services in 2002 for women with type 1 and type 2 diabetes in England, Wales and Northern Ireland.* CEMACH: London; 2004.

2. *Confidential Enquiry into Maternal and Child Health. Pregnancy in women with type 1 and type 2 diabetes in 2002-03, England, Wales and Northern Ireland.* CEMACH: London; 2005.

3. *"The Global Criteria for the WHO/UNICEF Baby-Friendly Hospital Initiative."* UNICEF. New York 1992.

4. Macfarlane A, Mungford M. *Birth Counts: Statistics of pregnancy and childbirth.* 2nd ed. Oxford: National Perinatal Epidemiology Unit; 2000.

5. *Care Recommendation: Recommendations for the management of pregnant women with diabetes (including Gestational diabetes).* Diabetes UK 2005.

6. *Management of Diabetes.* Scottish Intercollegiate Guidelines Network. 2001. SIGN Publication No.55. Edinburgh: SIGN.

7. *National Service Framework for Diabetes (England) Standards.* Department of Health. The Stationery Office; London; 2001.

8. Broadfoot M, Britten J, Tappin DM, Mackenzie JM. *The Baby Friendly Hospital Initiative and breast feeding rates in Scotland.* Arch Dis Child Fetal Neonatal Ed 2005; 90(2):F114-F116.

9. Kramer MS, Chalmers B, Hodnett ED, et al. *Promotion of breastfeeding intervention trial (PROBIT).* JAMA 2001; 285(January 24/31):413-420.

10. Levy-Shiff R, Lerman M, Har-Even D, Hod M. *Maternal adjustment and infant outcome in medically defined high-risk pregnancy.* Dev Psychol. 2002 Jan;38(1):93-103.

11. Christensson K, Siles C, Moreno L, Belaustequi A, De La Fuente P, Lagercrantz H, Puyol P, Winberg J. *Temperature, metabolic adaptation and crying in healthy full-term newborns cared for skin-to-skin or in a cot.* Acta Paediatr. 1992 Jun-Jul;81(6-7):488-93.

12. Christensson K, Cabrera T, Christensson E, Uvnas-Moberg K, Winberg J. *Separation distress call in the human neonate in the absence of maternal body contact.* Acta Paediatr. 1995 May;84(5):468-73.

13. Anderson GC, Moore E, Hepworth J, Bergman N. *Early skin-to-skin contact for mothers and their healthy newborn infants.* Cochrane Database Syst Rev. 2003;(2):CD003519.

14. Williams AF. *Hypoglycaemia of the newborn. Review of the literature.* World Health Organisation, Geneva 1997.

15. Hawdon JM, Ward Platt MP, Aynsley-Green A. *Patterns of metabolic adaptation for preterm and term infants in the first neonatal week.* Arch Dis Child 1992; 67:357-65.

16. *Infant feeding survey 2000.* The Stationery Office: London; 2002.

17. Deshpande S, Ward Platt M. *The investigation and management of neonatal hypoglycaemia. Seminars in Fetal & Neonatal Medicine (2005).* 10, 351-361.

18. de Rooy L, Hawdon *Nutritional factors that affect the postnatal metabolic adaptation of full-term small- and large-for-gestational-age infants.* J. Pediatrics 2002 Mar;109 (3): E42.

19. Ellis M, Manandhar DS, Manandhar N, Land JM, Patel N, de L Costello AM. *Comparison of two cotside methods for the detection of hypoglycaemia among neonates in Nepal.* Arch Dis Child Fetal Neonatal Ed 1996 Sep; 75(2):F122-5.

20. Dahlberg M, Whitelaw A. *Evaluation of HemoCue Blood Glucose Analyzer for the instant diagnosis of hypoglycaemia in newborns.* Scand J Clin Lab Invest 1997 Dec; 57(8):719-24.

21. Deshpande SA, Matthews JN, Platt MP. *Measuring blood glucose in neonatal units: how does hemocue compare?* Arch Dis Child Fetal Neonatal Ed. 1996 Nov;75(3):F202-8.

External commentary

Patricia Hamilton
President, Royal College of Paediatrics and Child Health

I welcome this important study conducted by CEMACH, and in particular their findings relating to the babies of women with diabetes. This work confirms what many have suspected, namely that the babies of women with diabetes are being admitted needlessly to neonatal units. Not only is there unnecessary separation from the mother, but also this inevitably has a negative impact on the success of breastfeeding. These two findings are against all the principles of child-friendly hospitals that we are trying to endorse and implement, and we hope that as a result of this report we can encourage more babies to remain with their mothers and achieve a higher success rate for breastfeeding.

This having been said, there is also concern regarding the sub-standard neonatal management of hypoglycaemia, as well as early feeding. With the best of intentions, junior trainees have been making estimates of blood glucose concentrations in babies too early and acting unnecessarily at a time when the baby's metabolism has not yet adjusted to extra uterine life and a low blood glucose concentration may be physiological. We hope that as a result of this report this practice will be improved.

CEMACH are to be congratulated on this careful piece of work, which will have practical implications for the betterment of the health of mothers and their babies.

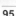

13. Conclusions

The St. Vincent declaration in 1989[1] that 'in five years, the outcome of diabetic pregnancy should approximate that of non-diabetic pregnancy', has not yet been achieved. However, there have been a number of national and local initiatives focusing on improving the care and outcomes of pregnant women with type 1 and type 2 diabetes.

The Diabetes National Service Framework [2], first published by the Department of Health in 2001, set out a series of national standards for the care of people with diabetes. This included a standard for pregnancy which emphasised the importance of tight blood glucose control before conception and during pregnancy in order to optimise the chance of a good pregnancy outcome. The NSF includes key interventions, targets and illustrative service models which are available for NHS organisations to draw upon during the development of their local services, and local NHS performance will be assessed against the three-year and ten-year targets in the NSF's Delivery Strategy.[3] In addition, the Diabetes Commissioning Toolkit[4] published by the Department of Health in November 2006 includes best practice quality markers, evidence of improvement, and key outcomes that should be sought by commissioners of services. In particular, it specifies that there should be evidence of defined leadership within specialist services and integration between primary and secondary care for pre-pregnancy care and support.

The CEMACH Diabetes Programme has provided a comprehensive national overview of diabetes maternity services, standards of care for women with diabetes, and the possible reasons underlying suboptimal clinical care and lack of involvement of women in their own care. This should aid health care providers and commissioners in planning the most appropriate services for their local populations. The programme has highlighted a number of areas which need to be addressed. These include poor preparation for pregnancy and the need for effective education programmes for women of childbearing age with diabetes; fragmented preconception care services and variations in the standard of preconception care provided by health professionals; the increasing problem of women with type 2 diabetes and their different needs; and neonatal care policies.

As a response to the finding that the majority of women with diabetes are poorly prepared for pregnancy, CEMACH, together with the Royal College of General Practitioners and Diabetes UK, has published a joint information leaflet for GPs and the primary care team. This sets out information about the appropriate care and advice to provide for women of childbearing age with diabetes. The leaflet has been distributed to GPs throughout the UK and is also available for downloading from the CEMACH website.

Poor preparation for pregnancy appears to be the next barrier to overcome for women with diabetes. The CEMACH programme has found that pregnant women with type 2 diabetes, who are also more likely to be from a Black, Asian and Other ethnic minority group and live in a deprived area, appear to be less likely to access preconception care and annual diabetes reviews than women with type 1 diabetes. In order to better understand the reasons and possible solutions to this, CEMACH has commenced a research project with the University College London (UCL) Elizabeth Garrett Anderson Institute for Women's Health which is funded by Novo Nordisk. This will investigate the issues affecting preconception care in women with type 1 and type 2 diabetes.

It is clear that commissioners and providers of health care in both primary and secondary care settings need to work collaboratively. Their joint aim should be to ensure that women with diabetes are better informed and motivated to manage their diabetes before they become pregnant and that accessible multidisciplinary services are provided for them before pregnancy, during pregnancy and after delivery.

References

1. *Workshop Report. Diabetes Care and Research in Europe: The Saint Vincent Declaration.* Diabetic Med 1990:7;360.
2. *Department of Health. National Service Framework for Diabetes (England) Standards.* London: The Stationery Office: 2001.
3. *Department of Health. National Service Framework for Diabetes: Delivery Strategy.* London: Department of Health: 2002 [http://www.dh.gov.uk/assetRoot/04/03/28/23/04032823.pdf] accessed 17 January 2007.
4. *Department of Health. Diabetes Commissioning Toolkit.* London: Department of Health. 2006 [http://www.dh.gov.uk/assetRoot/04/14/02/85/04140285.pdf] accessed 17 January 2007.

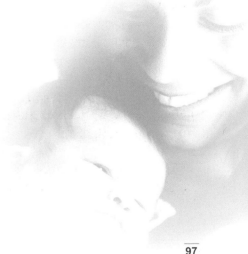

Appendix A: Pre-pregnancy care pro forma

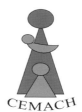

CONFIDENTIAL ENQUIRY INTO MATERNAL AND CHILD HEALTH

Diabetes Enquiry: Pre-pregnancy care pro forma

Woman's name: . . . .
(Forename, Surname)

Date of birth: . . . .
(dd/mm/yy)

Pregnancy dates: . . . .
(LMP to delivery/outcome date)

Please complete the following questions using information contemporaneous with the 12 month period prior to the above pregnancy

GENERAL INFORMATION

1. **Type of diabetes** ☐ Type 1 ☐ Type 2

2. **Was the woman's preferred language English?** ☐ Yes ☐ No ☐ Not documented

   If no, please specify preferred language: . . . .

   Was an interpreter provided by the service? ☐ Yes ☐ No ☐ Not documented

3. **Maternal height** (specify units) Height . . . . ☐ Not documented

4. **Pre-pregnancy weight** (specify units) Weight . . . . ☐ Not documented

5. **Did the woman smoke?** ☐ Yes ☐ No ☐ Not documented

   If yes, was she referred to a smoking cessation programme? ☐ Yes ☐ No ☐ Not documented

6. **Was the current pregnancy planned?** ☐ Yes ☐ No ☐ Not documented

7. **Was contraception being used prior to pregnancy?** ☐ Yes ☐ No ☐ Not documented

continued overleaf

Diabetes Enquiry: Pre-pregnancy care pro forma page 1

**CONFIDENTIAL ENQUIRY INTO
MATERNAL AND CHILD HEALTH**

8. Was contraceptive advice given prior to
   this pregnancy?
   ☐ Yes   ☐ No   ☐ Not documented

9. How many diabetic clinic appointments in
   the 12 month period prior to pregnancy did
   the woman have ?
   ☐☐ Appointment(s)   ☐ Not documented

10. How many of the above did she NOT ATTEND?
    ☐☐ Appointment(s)   ☐ Not documented

PRE-PREGNANCY REVIEW

11. Were the following issues specifically discussed
    with the woman prior to pregnancy?

    i.   alcohol intake   ☐ Yes   ☐ No   ☐ Not documented

    ii. diet   ☐ Yes   ☐ No   ☐ Not documented

    iii. poor glycaemic control   ☐ Yes   ☐ No   ☐ Not documented

    iv. retinopathy   ☐ Yes   ☐ No   ☐ Not documented

    v.   nephropathy   ☐ Yes   ☐ No   ☐ Not documented

    vi. hypertension   ☐ Yes   ☐ No   ☐ Not documented

12. Were any of the following tests carried out
    within 12 months of the LMP?

    i.   baseline retinal examination   ☐ Yes   ☐ No   ☐ Not documented

    ii. baseline renal function test i.e. U/E, Creatinine   ☐ Yes   ☐ No   ☐ Not documented

    iii. assessment of albuminuria   ☐ Yes   ☐ No   ☐ Not documented

13. Was there evidence of any diabetic complications
    in the 12 months prior to pregnancy?
    ☐ Yes   ☐ No   ☐ Not documented

    If yes, please describe . . . .
    . . . .

14. Was there evidence of any other medical or surgical
    complications in the 12 months prior to pregnancy?
    ☐ Yes   ☐ No   ☐ Not documented

    If yes, please describe . . . .
    . . . .

**CONFIDENTIAL ENQUIRY INTO
MATERNAL AND CHILD HEALTH**

15. Were the following elements of diabetic maternity care discussed with the woman?

i.	increased diabetic surveillance	☐ Yes ☐ No	☐ Not documented
ii.	increased pregnancy surveillance and scanning	☐ Yes ☐ No	☐ Not documented
iii.	increased risk of induction	☐ Yes ☐ No	☐ Not documented
iv.	possible delivery by caesarean section	☐ Yes ☐ No	☐ Not documented
v.	fetal risks in diabetic pregnancy (macrosomia, IUGR, congenital malformation)	☐ Yes ☐ No	☐ Not documented

16. Was the woman reviewed by a dietician?   ☐ Yes ☐ No ☐ Not documented

17. Was folic acid started prior to conception?   ☐ Yes ☐ No ☐ Not documented

If yes, date started (dd/mm/yy):   ☐☐/☐☐/☐☐

Dose of folic acid   ☐ 400mcg ☐ 5mg

☐ Other (specify) . . . .

18. Was pre-pregnancy care predominately carried out at:

☐ Hospital multidisciplinary clinic

☐ Hospital diabetes clinic

☐ GP surgery

☐ Other (specify) . . . .

Is the person completing this pro forma directly involved in the above clinic?   ☐ Yes ☐ No

---

PRE-PREGNANCY GLYCAEMIC CONTROL

19. Was a test done for glycaemic control before the LMP?   ☐ Yes ☐ No ☐ Not documented

	Date of test	Test result	Units	Laboratory range
If yes:	. . . .	. . . .	. . . .	. . . .

Type of test   ☐ Glycolated haemoglobin   ☐ Fructosamine   ☐ Other (specify) . . . .

20. Were specific targets set for pre-pregnancy glucose control and HbA1c?   ☐ Yes ☐ No ☐ Not documented

If yes, what was the target? (specify units)   . . . .

continued overleaf

Diabetes Enquiry: Pre-pregnancy care pro forma   Page 3

21. **Did this woman achieve the target HbA1c prior to becoming pregnant?**

☐ Yes ☐ No ☐ Not documented

22. **For women with type 2 diabetes only**

    i. Was this woman previously on oral agents?

    ☐ Yes ☐ No ☐ Not documented

    ii. What oral agents were used?

    Type | Dose

    . . . . | . . . .

    . . . . | . . . .

    . . . . | . . . .

    ☐ Not documented

    iii. Was transfer to insulin therapy undertaken prior to pregnancy?

    ☐ Yes ☐ No ☐ Not documented

Profession of person completing form . . . .

Completed by: . . . .

Date: . . . .

Contact tel. number: . . . .

The completed questionnaire should be returned to the CEMACH Regional Manager, as below:

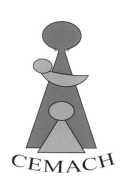

Confidential Enquiry into Maternal and Child Health

Improving health for mothers, babies and children

Diabetes enquiry pro forma

Do not keep any duplicates or copies of this form
Do not enter any names or signatures

Enquiry reference number:

_____

Panel members:
Mark box as appropriate
Enter a number into box if several members from one specialty

Obstetric	☐	Neonatal nursing	☐
Midwifery	☐	Diabetologist	☐
Neonatology	☐	Diabetic nurse specialist	☐
Lay representative	☐		

Other, specify: _____

_____

Confidential Enquiry into Maternal and Child Health
Improving health for mothers, babies and children

Guidance for completing the pro forma

Please read before proceeding to complete this assessment

Panel Guidance

Some questions in the enquiry pro forma include guidance (in italics) for the panel assessors. The purpose of this guidance is to aid consistent definitions and is not intended to be prescriptive. This is particularly relevant when evaluating glycaemic control as it is recognised that the panel may have access to information at enquiry which is at variance with the guidance provided. In this situation it is expected that the panel will make a decision based on all the information available rather than on the guidance only.

Terminations and Intrauterine Death

Only the relevant sections need be completed. We have a record of both the pregnancy outcome and gestation so all subsequent questions can be automatically coded as not applicable in analysis.

'No' and 'Not Documented' options

Only use the 'no' option where it is documented in the notes that something has not been done or is not present. We are aware that the nature of note keeping makes the 'no' option redundant in many questions but we need to record the information in this way for consistency in analysis. Use the 'not documented' option in all other situations.

Coding

The intention with the diabetes enquiry pro forma is that where glycaemic control, clinical care or the woman's approach to managing her diabetes is thought to be poor or adequate, the qualitative issues that informed this decision should be précised in the accompanying free text space. However in order to assist us with analysis of the data at a later stage there is also a basic coding system in operation. This means that wherever possible the free text should be categorised into main and supplementary codes by the panel as below. It is not essential to provide supplementary codes so please only complete if appropriate. We are aware that the codes are simplistic and that cases reviewed at panel are often complex with multiple issues, but the intention is only to assist in analysis and the detail of the free text will always be studied.

Broadly there are two categories of codes, those relating to the woman and her diabetes and those relating to the provision of health services.

A prefix **P** denotes that the issues discussed relate directly to the patient and/or family issues and the codes are:

> **PD** Duration or severity of diabetes
> **PO** Other complicating medical or social and/or lifestyle factors which may hinder optimal management e.g. management-intensive medical conditions such as thrombophilia or cardiac disease, and social factors such as housing problems or lack of family support
> **PC** Woman actively chose not to follow the medical advice given e.g. refusal to undergo induction of labour until 42+ weeks of gestation
> **PA** Woman's actions detracted from optimal management e.g. infrequent home blood glucose monitoring, not following dietary instructions
> **PN** Woman did not attend appointments e.g. failure to attend for clinic visits or ultrasound scans

A prefix **H** denotes that the issues discussed relate to the provision of health services and the codes are:

> **HP** Clinical practice e.g. no timely discussion of timing and mode of delivery
> **HC** Communication. This could be a failure of communication between professionals caring for the woman e.g. inadequate discussion between obstetrician and physician or a failure of communication between professionals and the woman e.g. interpreting services were not adequate despite difficulties with English
> **HR** Resources including staffing e.g. no dietician in the antenatal clinic, lack of midwifery staff on labour ward, problems with accessing timely fetal surveillance such as growth scans

Confidential Enquiry into Maternal and Child Health
Improving health for mothers, babies and children

CEMACH

PRE-PREGNANCY CARE *Please complete with reference to the pre-pregnancy pro forma*

1. **Does the panel think the woman's glycaemic control was optimal, adequate or poor prior to conception?**
   (Panel guidance: HbA1c<7% optimal, 7 to 8% adequate, >8% poor but please consider all available information including home blood glucose testing results and episodes of hypoglycaemia when making an assessment)

   ☐ Optimal

   ☐ Adequate

   ☐ Poor

   ☐ Insufficient information in notes

   If poor or adequate, please summarise key issues and code accordingly:

   _____

   _____

   _____

   _____

   ☐☐ Main code   ☐☐ Supplementary codes
                          ☐☐
                          ☐☐

2. **Does the panel think pre-pregnancy care, other than glycaemic control, was optimal, adequate or poor?**
   (Panel guidance: please consider the assessment and treatment of complications, advice given, folic acid and other information contained in the pre-pregnancy pro forma. Optimal indicates that there are no issues with care that need documenting, adequate indicates that there are some issues)

   ☐ Optimal

   ☐ Adequate

   ☐ Poor

   ☐ Insufficient information in notes

   If poor or adequate, please summarise key issues and code accordingly:

   _____

   _____

   _____

   _____

   ☐☐ Main code   ☐☐ Supplementary codes
                          ☐☐
                          ☐☐

Diabetes enquiry pro forma   Page 3

Confidential Enquiry into Maternal and Child Health
Improving health for mothers, babies and children

PREGNANCY CARE (up to delivery)

3. **Was the current pregnancy planned?** ☐ Yes ☐ No ☐ Not documented

4. **Was this woman a primagravida?** ☐ Yes ☐ No ☐ Not documented

   a) If no, please indicate if any previous pregnancy ended in a congenital malformation ☐ Yes ☐ No ☐ Not documented

5. **Did this woman have gestational diabetes in a previous pregnancy?**
   (only complete if woman has Type 2 diabetes) ☐ Yes ☐ No ☐ Not documented
   ☐ Not applicable

6. **What was the date at first contact with a health professional this pregnancy? (dd/mm/yy)** ☐☐/☐☐/☐☐

7. **What was the date at first hospital appointment this pregnancy? (dd/mm/yy)** ☐☐/☐☐/☐☐

8. **Please indicate which professionals were involved in the antenatal care of this woman:**

   ☐ physician ☐ midwife with special interest in diabetes ☐ diabetes nurse specialist

   ☐ dietician ☐ obstetrician with special interest in diabetes

9. **Was antenatal care carried out in a dedicated multidisciplinary combined clinic?**
   (Panel guidance: a clinic where the relevant professionals are present at the same time) ☐ Yes ☐ No ☐ Not documented

10. **Was a retinal assessment performed in the first trimester or at booking if later?** ☐ Yes ☐ No ☐ Not documented

    a) If yes, was this through dilated pupils? ☐ Yes ☐ No ☐ Not documented

11. **Was retinopathy present?** ☐ Yes ☐ No ☐ Not documented

    If yes, please answer a) and b)

    a) Please indicate type: ☐ Pre-existing – no change ☐ Pre-existing and deteriorating
    ☐ New finding

    b) Was the woman referred to an ophthalmologist? ☐ Yes ☐ No ☐ Not documented

12. **Was folic acid taken in the first trimester?** ☐ Yes ☐ No ☐ Not documented

    If yes, please answer a) and b)

    a) Please specify dose of folic acid ☐ 400mcg ☐ 4-5mg ☐ Dose not specified

    b) Please indicate when folic acid started (completed weeks) ☐☐

Confidential Enquiry into Maternal and Child Health
Improving health for mothers, babies and children

| | PREGNANCY CARE (up to delivery) continued |

13. Was this woman monitored for signs of nephropathy? ☐ Yes ☐ No ☐ Not documented

14. Did this woman have diabetic nephropathy? ☐ Yes ☐ No ☐ Not documented

If yes, please answer a) and b)

a) Please indicate type: ☐ Incipient with microalbuminuria

☐ Established with persistent dip stick positive proteinuria and/or serum creatinine>130

b) Was renal function monitored adequately? ☐ Yes ☐ No ☐ Not documented
(Panel guidance: at least every trimester by 24 hour urinary protein estimation in women with microalbuminuria. At least monthly monitoring of urine and blood in women with macro-proteinuria)

15. Were there recurrent episodes of hypoglycaemia during pregnancy? ☐ Yes ☐ No ☐ Not documented

16. Did any episode of hypoglycaemia require help from another person? ☐ Yes ☐ No ☐ Not documented

17. Were there any pre-existing diabetic complications that required treatment during the last year? ☐ Yes ☐ No ☐ Not documented

If yes, please describe:

_____

_____

_____

18. Were there any other medical or surgical complications that required treatment during the last year? ☐ Yes ☐ No ☐ Not documented

If yes, please describe:

_____

_____

_____

19. Was a target range set for blood glucose control during the first trimester (prior to 13 weeks)? ☐ Yes ☐ No ☐ Not documented
(Panel guidance: if not documented in the notes but included in the hospital protocol please complete as yes)

a) If yes, was this target range communicated to the woman? ☐ Yes ☐ No ☐ Not documented

Diabetes enquiry pro forma Page 5

Confidential Enquiry into Maternal and Child Health
Improving health for mothers, babies and children

	PREGNANCY CARE (up to delivery) continued

20. Was a target range set for blood glucose control thereafter (from 13 weeks up to labour and delivery)?
(Panel guidance: if not documented in the notes but included in the hospital protocol please complete as yes)

☐ Yes   ☐ No   ☐ Not documented

☐ Not applicable

a) If yes, was this target range communicated to the woman?

☐ Yes   ☐ No   ☐ Not documented

21. Does the panel think the woman's glycaemic control was optimal, adequate or poor:
(Panel guidance: HbA1c<7% optimal, 7 to 8% adequate, >8% poor)

a) In the first trimester (prior to 13 weeks)?

☐ Optimal

☐ Adequate

☐ Poor

☐ Insufficient information in notes

If poor or adequate, please summarise key issues and code accordingly:

_____

_____

_____

_____

☐☐ Main code   ☐☐ Supplementary codes

                       ☐☐

                       ☐☐

b) Thereafter (from 13 weeks up to labour and delivery)?

☐ Optimal

☐ Adequate

☐ Poor

☐ Insufficient information in notes

If poor or adequate, please summarise key issues and code accordingly:

_____

_____

_____

_____

☐☐ Main code   ☐☐ Supplementary codes

                       ☐☐

                       ☐☐

Confidential Enquiry into Maternal and Child Health
Improving health for mothers, babies and children

PREGNANCY CARE (up to delivery) continued

22. Does the panel think the diabetic care of the mother during pregnancy, other than glycaemic control, was optimal, adequate or poor? *(Panel guidance: Please consider retinal & renal screening and the management of any complications. Optimal indicates that there are no issues with care that need documenting, adequate indicates that there are some issues)*

☐ Optimal

☐ Adequate

☐ Poor

☐ Insufficient information in notes

If poor or adequate, please summarise key issues and code accordingly:

_____

_____

_____

_____

☐☐ Main code   ☐☐ Supplementary codes
                      ☐☐
                      ☐☐

23. Does the panel think the maternity care of the mother during pregnancy was optimal, adequate or poor?
(Panel guidance: optimal indicates that there are no issues with care that need documenting, adequate indicates that there are some issues)

☐ Optimal

☐ Adequate

☐ Poor

☐ Insufficient information in notes

If poor or adequate, please summarise key issues and code accordingly:

_____

_____

_____

_____

☐☐ Main code   ☐☐ Supplementary codes
                      ☐☐
                      ☐☐

Confidential Enquiry into Maternal and Child Health
Improving health for mothers, babies and children

FETAL ASSESSMENT (before labour)

24. Was there antenatal evidence of:

a) Fetal growth restriction or poor growth velocity? ☐ Yes ☐ No ☐ Not documented

b) Fetal size greater than 90th centile? ☐ Yes ☐ No ☐ Not documented

c) If yes to either a) or b), does the panel think the subsequent monitoring of fetal well being was optimal, adequate or poor? *(Panel guidance: optimal indicates that there are no issues with care that need documenting, adequate indicates that there are some issues)*

☐ Optimal

☐ Adequate

☐ Poor

☐ Insufficient information in notes

If poor or adequate, please summarise key issues and code accordingly:

_____

_____

_____

☐☐ Main code   ☐☐ Supplementary codes
                 ☐☐
                 ☐☐

LABOUR AND DELIVERY

25. What was the date of delivery? (dd/mm/yy)   ☐☐/☐☐/☐☐

26. Was this delivery less than 36^{+0} weeks? ☐ Yes ☐ No ☐ Not documented
                                                          ☐ Not applicable

If yes:
a) Were any corticosteroids given? ☐ Yes ☐ No ☐ Not documented

b) If corticosteroids were not given, please give reason if documented:

_____

_____

_____

_____

Confidential Enquiry into Maternal and Child Health
Improving health for mothers, babies and children

CEMACH

LABOUR AND DELIVERY continued

c) If corticosteroids were given, were any of the following undertaken:

i. Increased checking of blood glucose? ☐ Yes ☐ No ☐ Not documented

ii. Change in subcutaneous insulin regime? ☐ Yes ☐ No ☐ Not documented

iii. Intravenous dextrose and insulin? ☐ Yes ☐ No ☐ Not documented

27. **Was the mode and timing of delivery discussed with the woman?** ☐ Yes ☐ No ☐ Not documented
☐ Not applicable

a) If yes, at what gestation was this first discussed (completed weeks)? ☐☐

28. **Were intravenous dextrose and insulin administered during labour and delivery?** ☐ Yes ☐ No ☐ Not documented
☐ Not applicable

If no, give any documented reason:

_____

_____

29. **Was a target range set for blood glucose control during labour and delivery?** *(Panel guidance: if not documented in the notes but included in the hospital protocol please complete as yes)* ☐ Yes ☐ No ☐ Not documented
☐ Not applicable

30. **Does the panel think the management of the woman's blood glucose control was optimal, adequate or poor during labour and delivery?** *(Panel guidance: 3.5 to 8 mmols/l optimal, 8 to 9 adequate, > 9 poor)*

☐ Optimal   ☐ Not applicable

☐ Adequate

☐ Poor

☐ Insufficient information in notes

If poor or adequate, please summarise key issues and code accordingly:

_____

_____

_____

_____

☐☐ Main code   ☐☐ Supplementary codes
☐☐
☐☐

Diabetes enquiry pro forma   Page 9

Confidential Enquiry into Maternal and Child Health
Improving health for mothers, babies and children

31. Does the panel think that maternity care during labour and delivery was optimal, adequate or poor?
(Panel guidance: optimal indicates that there are no issues with care that need documenting, adequate indicates that there are some issues)

☐ Optimal   ☐ Not applicable

☐ Adequate

☐ Poor

☐ Insufficient information in notes

If poor or adequate, please summarise key issues and code accordingly:

_____

_____

_____

_____

☐☐ Main code   ☐☐ Supplementary codes

                                    ☐☐

                                    ☐☐

POSTNATAL CARE OF MOTHER

32. Was there a plan for post delivery diabetic management while still in hospital?   ☐ Yes   ☐ No   ☐ Not documented   ☐ Not applicable

33. Was contraceptive advice given prior to discharge from hospital?   ☐ Yes   ☐ No   ☐ Not documented   ☐ Not applicable

34. Was there a follow-up appointment for diabetic management arranged prior to discharge from hospital?   ☐ Yes   ☐ No   ☐ Not documented   ☐ Not applicable

35. Does the panel think postnatal diabetic care and advice was optimal, adequate or poor? *(Panel guidance: optimal indicates that there are no issues with care that need documenting, adequate indicates that there are some issues)*

☐ Optimal   ☐ Not applicable

☐ Adequate

☐ Poor

Confidential Enquiry into Maternal and Child Health
Improving health for mothers, babies and children

POSTNATAL CARE OF MOTHER continued

If poor or adequate, please summarise key issues and code accordingly:

_____

_____

_____

_____

[ ][ ] Main code   [ ][ ] Supplementary codes
                          [ ][ ]
                          [ ][ ]

NEONATAL CARE

36. **Was the baby separated from its mother after delivery?**   ☐ Yes ☐ No ☐ Not documented ☐ Not applicable

If yes please give the reason for this:

_____

_____

_____

37. **Was there an intended method of feeding in notes?**   ☐ Yes ☐ No ☐ Not documented ☐ Not applicable

38. **Was supplemental milk or glucose given in the first 24 hours after delivery?**   ☐ Yes ☐ No ☐ Not documented ☐ Not applicable

39. **Was low reagent stick measurement (<2.6mmol/l) checked by laboratory examination?**   ☐ Yes ☐ No ☐ Not documented ☐ Not applicable

Please give method:

_____

_____

_____

_____

Confidential Enquiry into Maternal and Child Health
Improving health for mothers, babies and children

PATHOLOGY

40. Was placental pathology carried out? ☐ Yes ☐ No ☐ Not documented

If yes, please indicate whether any of the following were found:

a) Cord oedema ☐ Yes ☐ No ☐ Not documented

b) Villious oedema ☐ Yes ☐ No ☐ Not documented

c) Villious immaturity ☐ Yes ☐ No ☐ Not documented

Please specify any further relevant finding:

_____

_____

_____

CONGENITAL MALFORMATION (only complete if baby has congenital malformation) ☐ Not applicable

41. When was the congenital malformation first detected?

☐ antenatally

☐☐ Please give gestation (completed weeks)

☐ postnatally

42. Was the congenital malformation confirmed? ☐ Yes ☐ No ☐ Not documented

If yes, please give method of confirmation:

_____

_____

_____

POST MORTEM (only complete if baby died) ☐ Not applicable

43. Was a post mortem offered? ☐ Yes ☐ No ☐ Not documented

44. Was a post mortem carried out? ☐ Yes ☐ No ☐ Not documented

If no, please give reason:

_____

_____

_____

_____

Confidential Enquiry into Maternal and Child Health
Improving health for mothers, babies and children

CEMACH

	POST MORTEM continued

45. Was the post mortem report available at panel? ☐ Yes ☐ No ☐ Not documented

If yes, please indicate whether any of the following were found:

a) Pancreas: Islet Cell hyperplasia ☐ Yes ☐ No ☐ Not documented

Eosinophilic pancreatitis ☐ Yes ☐ No ☐ Not documented

b) Heart: Cardiomegaly/fibre disarray ☐ Yes ☐ No ☐ Not documented

c) Kidneys: Vascular thrombosis ☐ Yes ☐ No ☐ Not documented

Please specify any further relevant finding:

_____

_____

_____

_____

Please go to summary section on the next page

Confidential Enquiry into Maternal and Child Health
Improving health for mothers, babies and children

CEMACH

SUMMARY SECTION

46. **Does the panel think that the overall diabetes care was optimal, adequate or poor?** *(Panel guidance: this is a summary of glycaemic control and other aspects of diabetic care from preconception through to the postnatal period. Detailed issues should be documented earlier in the pro forma)*

☐ Optimal

☐ Adequate

☐ Poor

☐ Insufficient information in notes

47. **Does the panel think that the overall maternity care was optimal, adequate or poor?** *(Panel guidance: this is a summary of maternity care throughout pregnancy. Detailed issues should be documented earlier in the pro forma)*

☐ Optimal

☐ Adequate

☐ Poor

☐ Insufficient information in notes

48. **Does the panel think the woman's approach to managing her diabetes was optimal, adequate or poor:**

   a) In the preconception period? *(Panel guidance: optimal indicates that there are no issues that need documenting, adequate indicates that there are some issues)*

☐ Optimal

☐ Adequate

☐ Poor

☐ Insufficient information in notes

If poor or adequate, please summarise key issues and code accordingly:

_____

_____

_____

_____

☐☐ Main code   ☐☐ Supplementary codes
                          ☐☐
                          ☐☐

Confidential Enquiry into Maternal and Child Health
Improving health for mothers, babies and children

CEMACH

SUMMARY SECTION continued

b)   During pregnancy? (*Panel guidance: optimal indicates that there are no issues that need documenting, adequate indicates that there are some issues*)

☐ Optimal

☐ Adequate

☐ Poor

☐ Insufficient information in notes

If poor or adequate, please summarise key issues and code accordingly:

_____

_____

_____

_____

☐☐ Main code   ☐☐ Supplementary codes
                       ☐☐
                       ☐☐

49. Does the panel think there were any deficiencies in communication between the different professionals involved in the woman's care?   ☐ Yes   ☐ No   ☐ Not possible to infer from notes

If yes, please summarise key issues detailing disciplines involved and grades:

_____

_____

_____

_____

50. Does the panel think there were any deficiencies in communication with the woman?   ☐ Yes   ☐ No   ☐ Not possible to infer from notes

If yes, please summarise key issues detailing both the professionals' and woman's contribution:

_____

_____

_____

_____

Diabetes enquiry pro forma   Page 15

Confidential Enquiry into Maternal and Child Health
Improving health for mothers, babies and children

51. Does the panel think there were any deficiencies in the standard of notes? *(Panel guidance: please comment on whether this is to do with the structure of notes or quality of note keeping)*

   a)   obstetric notes   ☐ Yes   ☐ No

   If yes, please comment:

_____

_____

_____

   b)   diabetic notes   ☐ Yes   ☐ No

   If yes, please comment:

_____

_____

_____

_____

52. Does the panel think there were any deficiencies in the hospital protocols?   ☐ Yes   ☐ No   ☐ Not available at panel meeting

   If yes, please comment:

_____

_____

_____

Diabetes enquiry pro forma

Confidential Enquiry into Maternal and Child Health
Improving health for mothers, babies and children

CEMACH

SUMMARY SECTION continued

53. Please add any additional relevant information or comments not captured elsewhere on the pro forma.

54. Please list any examples of good practice that you think should be shared.

Confidential Enquiry into Maternal and Child Health
Improving health for mothers, babies and children

For completion by Panel Chair and Regional Manager after enquiry.

55. **Please note any positive or negative issues relating to the 3 areas defined below. This will help to evaluate the panel enquiry process and make improvements for further enquiry work.**

    a) Panel Process:

    b) Lay member/s involvement in the panel meeting:

    c) Clinical issues noted during panel enquiry (e.g. inconsistency of existing definitions, variance in practice):

Appendix C

Association between demographic and clinical characteristics, social and lifestyle factors, and clinical care with major fetal congenital anomaly in the offspring of women with type 1 and type 2 diabetes

Association of demographic characteristics with major fetal congenital anomaly in the offspring of women with type 1 and type 2 diabetes				
Demographic characteristic	**Cases n/N (%)**	**Controls n/N (%)**	**Crude OR [95% CI]**	**Adjusted OR**
Age	-	-	1.0 [1.0, 1.1]	1.0 [1.0, 1.1][b]
Black, Asian or Other Ethnic Minority group	22/127 (17)	41/220 (19)	0.9 [0.5, 1.6]	0.6 [0.3, 1.2][a]
Primigravidity	52/127 (41)	92/220 (42)	1.0 [0.6, 1.5]	1.1 [0.7, 1.8][a]
Maternal social deprivation[d]	-	-	1.2 [1.0, 1.4]	1.2 [1.0, 1.4][c]

[a] adjusted for maternal age and deprivation.

[b] adjusted for maternal deprivation.

[c] adjusted for maternal age. Odds ratio is for one year increase in maternal age.

[d] Quintile of social deprivation derived from postcode of residence. Odds ratio is for unit increase in deprivation quintile.

Association of clinical characteristics with major fetal congenital anomaly in the offspring of women with type 1 and type 2 diabetes				
Clinical characteristic	**Cases n/N (%)**	**Controls n/N (%)**	**Crude OR [95% CI]**	**Adjusted OR[a]**
Body Mass Index (BMI ≥ 30)	53/80 (66)	33/137 (24)	1.6 [0.9, 3.0]	1.3 [0.7, 2.5]
Pre-existing diabetes complications	22/104 (21)	16/197 (8)	3.0 [1.5, 6.2]	3.1 [1.5, 6.3]
Retinopathy in pregnancy	34/88 (39)	50/167 (30)	1.5 [0.9, 2.5]	1.5 [0.9, 2.7]
Diabetic nephropathy in pregnancy	14/103 (13)	14/185 (8)	1.9 [0.9, 4.2]	1.7 [0.7, 3.9]
Recurrent episodes of hypoglycaemia during pregnancy	56/109 (51)	105/205 (51)	1.0 [0.6, 1.6]	1.1 [0.6, 1.8]
Severe hypoglycaemia during pregnancy (one or more episodes of hypoglycaemia requiring external help)	18/78 (23)	32/167 (19)	1.3 [0.7, 2.4]	1.4 [0.7, 2.8]
Antenatal evidence of fetal growth restriction	15/105 (14)	11/218 (5)	3.1 [1.4, 7.2]	3.0 [1.2, 7.0]
Antenatal evidence of macrosomia (fetal size >90th centile)	21/100 (21)	76/216 (35)	0.5 [0.3, 0.9]	0.5 [0.3, 0.9]

[a] adjusted for maternal age and deprivation.

Association of social and lifestyle factors with major fetal congenital anomaly in the offspring of women with type 1 and type 2 diabetes				
Social and lifestyle factor	Cases n/N (%)	Controls n/N (%)	Crude OR [95% CI]	Adjusted OR[a]
Unplanned pregnancy	43/75 (57)	55/144 (38)	2.2 [1.2, 3.9]	2.3 [1.3, 4.3]
No contraceptive use in the 12 months before pregnancy	33/55 (60)	54/121 (45)	1.9 [1.0, 3.6]	2.0 [1.0, 4.0]
No folic acid commenced prior to pregnancy	49/69 (71)	66/131 (50)	2.4 [1.3, 4.6]	2.3 [1.2, 4.5]
Smoking	35/103 (34)	44/182 (24)	1.6 [1.0, 2.8]	2.2 [1.2, 3.9]
Assessment of suboptimal approach of the woman to managing her diabetes before pregnancy	80/92 (86)	88/154 (57)	4.6 [2.3, 9.3]	5.0 [2.4, 10.2]
Assessment of suboptimal approach of the woman to managing her diabetes during pregnancy	62/110 (56)	56/207 (27)	3.5 [2.1, 5.8]	3.5 [2.0, 5.9]

[a] Adjusted for maternal age and deprivation

Association of glycaemic control factors before and during pregnancy with major fetal congenital anomaly in the offspring of women with type 1 and type 2 diabetes				
Glycaemic control factor	Cases n/N (%)	Controls n/N (%)	Crude OR [95% CI]	Adjusted OR[a]
No test of glycaemic control before pregnancy	18/76 (24)	24/139 (17)	1.5 [0.7, 3.0]	1.2 [0.6, 2.6]
No local targets set for glycaemic control	20/43 (47)	28/86 (33)	1.8 [0.8, 3.9]	1.8 [0.8, 4.1]
Assessment of suboptimal preconception glycaemic control	96/111 (86)	115/167 (69)	2.9 [1.5, 5.5]	3.6 [1.8, 7.2]
Assessment of suboptimal 1st trimester glycaemic control	94/115 (82)	118/192 (61)	2.8 [1.6, 4.0]	3.3 [1.8, 6.0]
Assessment of suboptimal glycaemic control after 1st trimester	78/112 (70)	76/209 (37)	4.0 [2.4, 6.8]	5.5 [3.2, 9.6]
Assessment of suboptimal blood glucose control during labour and delivery	38/92 (41)	94/202 (47)	0.8 [0.5, 1.3]	0.9 [0.5, 1.5]
No intravenous insulin and dextrose during labour and/or delivery	27/115 (23)	31/127 (14)	1.8 [1.0, 3.3]	1.8 [1.0, 3.3]

[a] Adjusted for maternal age and deprivation.

Association of preconception care factors in the 12 months prior to pregnancy with major fetal congenital anomaly in the offspring of women with type 1 and type 2 diabetes				
Preconception care factor	**Cases n/N (%)**	**Controls n/N (%)**	**Crude OR [95% CI]**	**Adjusted OR[a]**
No contraceptive advice provided before pregnancy	16/49 (33)	19/83 (23)	1.6 [0.7, 3.6]	1.6 [0.7, 3.8]
No discussion of the following specific diabetes issues:				
Alcohol	15/36 (42)	19/66 (29)	1.8 [0.8, 4.2]	2.2 [0.9, 5.7]
Diet	10/56 (18)	12/100 (12)	1.6 [0.6, 4.0]	1.6 [0.6, 4.2]
Poor glycaemic control	8/66 (12)	14/117 (12)	1.0 [0.4, 2.6]	0.8 [0.3, 2.2]
Retinopathy	11/50 (22)	25/96 (26)	0.8 [0.4, 1.8]	0.6 [0.3, 1.6]
Nephropathy	13/40 (33)	29/76 (38)	0.8 [0.4, 1.8]	0.5 [0.2, 1.4]
Hypertension	12/39 (31)	23/75 (31)	1.0 [0.4, 2.3]	0.6 [0.2, 1.7]
No discussion of the following pregnancy issues:				
Increased diabetes surveillance	5/61 (8)	7/124 (6)	1.5 [0.5, 4.9]	1.4 [0.4, 5.0]
Increased pregnancy surveillance	5/62 (8)	8/124 (6)	1.3 [0.4, 4.1]	1.2 [0.4, 4.0]
Increased risk of induction	10/43 (23)	14/110 (13)	2.1 [0.8, 5.2]	2.3 [0.9, 6.0]
Possible caesarean section	7/49 (14)	11/110 (10)	1.5 [0.5, 4.2]	1.8 [0.6, 5.2]
Fetal risks in diabetic pregnancy	7/52 (13)	7/114 (6)	2.4 [0.8, 7.3]	2.8 [0.8, 9.3]
No dietetic review	*24/69 (35)*	*42/135 (61)*	*1.2 [0.6, 2.2]*	*1.2 [0.6, 2.2]*
No assessment of the following diabetes complications in the 12 months prior to pregnancy:				
Baseline retinal examination	19/80 (24)	18/137 (13)	2.1 [1.0, 4.2]	2.0 [0.9, 4.4]
Baseline test of renal function	12/72 (17)	15/133 (11)	1.6 [0.7, 3.6]	1.6 [0.6, 3.9]
Assessment of albuminuria	22/62 (35)	30/109 (28)	1.5 [0.7, 2.8]	1.4 [0.7, 3.0]
Assessment of suboptimal preconception care (excluding glycaemic control)	68/75 (91)	80/134 (60)	6.6 [2.7, 16.2]	7.0 [2.9, 17.1]

[a] Adjusted for maternal age and deprivation.

Association of diabetes care factors (excluding glycaemic control) with major fetal congenital anomaly in the offspring of women with type 1 and type 2 diabetes				
Diabetes care factor	**Cases n/N (%)**	**Controls n/N (%)**	**Crude OR [95% CI]**	**Adjusted OR[a]**
No retinal assessment during 1st trimester or at booking if later	43/111 (39)	49/183 (27)	1.7 [1.0, 2.9]	1.5 [0.9, 2.6]
No referral to ophthalmologist (if retinopathy present)	4/29 (14)	21/44 (48)	0.2 [0.1, 0.6]	0.1 [0.0, 0.4]
No monitoring for nephropathy	27/118 (23)	26/206 (13)	2.1 [1.1, 3.8]	2.0 [1.1, 3.7]
No test of renal function (if nephropathy present)	4/12 (33)	5/14 (36)	0.9 [0.2, 4.7]	0.4 [0.1, 3.2]
Assessment of suboptimal diabetes care during pregnancy	74/113 (65)	112/204 (55)	1.6 [1.0, 2.5]	1.4 [0.9, 2.3]

[a] Adjusted for maternal age and deprivation.

Association of maternity care factors with major fetal congenital anomaly in the offspring of women with type 1 and type 2 diabetes				
Maternity care factor	**Cases n/N (%)**	**Controls n/N (%)**	**Crude OR [95% CI]**	**Adjusted OR[a]**
Assessment of suboptimal fetal monitoring (with antenatal evidence of growth restricted baby)	1/13 (8)	1/11 (9)	0.8 [0.0, 16.1]	0.4 [0.0, 8.0]
Assessment of suboptimal fetal monitoring (with antenatal evidence of fetal size >90th centile)	7/20 (35)	27/73 (37)	1.2 [0.4, 3.3]	1.1 [0.3, 3.7]
No discussion of mode and timing of delivery	6/102 (6)	4/202 (2)	3.1 [0.9, 11.3]	2.5 [0.6, 9.8]
No administration of antenatal corticosteroids[b]	12/34 (35)	12/33 (36)	1.0 [0.4, 2.6]	1.0 [0.3, 2.9]
Assessment of suboptimal maternity care during the antenatal period	57/125 (46)	95/215 (44)	1.1 [0.7, 1.7]	1.1 [0.7, 1.8]
Assessment of suboptimal maternity care during labour and delivery	44/111 (40)	72/213 (34)	1.3 [0.8, 2.1]	1.3 [0.8, 2.1]

[a] Adjusted for maternal age and deprivation.

[b] Analysis restricted to babies delivering from 24+0 to 35+6 weeks gestation and excluding antepartum stillbirths.

Association of postnatal care factors with major fetal congenital anomaly in the offspring of women with type 1 and type 2 diabetes				
Postnatal care factor	**Cases** n/N (%)	**Controls** n/N (%)	**Crude OR** [95% CI]	**Adjusted OR[a]**
No postnatal contraceptive advice	39/83 (47)	26/163 (16)	4.7 [2.5, 3.9]	4.3 [2.3, 8.2]
No written plan for post-delivery diabetes management	19/100 (19)	25/188 (13)	1.5 [0.8, 3.0]	1.8 [0.9, 3.5]
Assessment of suboptimal postnatal diabetes care	72/116 (62)	106/211 (50)	1.6 [1.0, 2.6]	1.4 [0.9, 2.3]

[a] Adjusted for maternal age and deprivation.

Appendix D

Association of demographic and clinical characteristics, social and lifestyle factors, and clinical care with all fetal and neonatal deaths from 20 weeks of gestation up to 28 days after delivery in babies of women with type 1 and type 2 diabetes

Association of demographic characteristics with fetal and neonatal death from 20 weeks gestation in babies of women with type 1 and type 2 diabetes				
Demographic characteristic	Cases n/N (%)	Controls n/N (%)	Crude OR [95% CI]	Adjusted OR
Age	-	-	1.0 [1.0, 1.0]	1.0 [1.0, 1.0][b]
Black, Asian or Other Ethnic Minority group	35/137 (26)	41/220 (19)	1.5 [0.9, 2.5]	1.2 [0.7, 2.2][a]
Primigravidity	65/137 (47)	92/220 (42)	1.3 [0.8, 1.9]	1.4 [0.9, 2.3][a]
Maternal social deprivation[d]	-	-	1.2 [1.0, 1.4]	1.2 [1.0, 1.4][c]

[a] adjusted for maternal age and deprivation.

[b] adjusted for maternal deprivation.

[c] adjusted for maternal age. Odds ratio is for one year increase in maternal age.

[d] Quintile of social deprivation derived from postcode of residence. Odds ratio is for unit increase in deprivation quintile.

Association of clinical characteristics with fetal and neonatal death from 20 weeks gestation in babies of women with type 1 and type 2 diabetes				
Clinical characteristic	Cases n/N (%)	Controls n/N (%)	Crude OR [95% CI]	Adjusted OR[a]
Body Mass Index (BMI ≥ 30)	22/81 (27)	33/137 (24)	1.2 [0.6, 2.2]	1.0 [0.5, 2.1]
Pre-existing diabetes complications	25/115 (22)	16/197 (8)	3.1 [1.6, 6.3]	2.7 [1.3, 5.5]
Retinopathy in pregnancy	32/89 (36)	50/167 (30)	1.3 [0.8, 2.3]	1.5 [0.0, 2.0]
Diabetic nephropathy in pregnancy	17/108 (16)	14/185 (8)	2.3 [1.1, 4.9]	2.0 [0.9, 4.5]
Recurrent episodes of hypoglycaemia during pregnancy	62/125 (50)	105/205 (51)	0.9 [0.6, 1.5]	1.1 [0.7, 1.8]
Severe hypoglycaemia during pregnancy (one or more episodes of hypoglycaemia requiring external help)	16/90 (18)	32/167 (19)	0.9 [0.5, 1.8]	1.0 [0.5, 2.1]
Antenatal evidence of fetal growth restriction	14/113 (12)	11/218 (5)	2.7 [1.2, 6.1]	2.6 [1.1, 6.2]
Antenatal evidence of macrosomia (fetal size >90th centile)	34/109 (31)	76/216 (35)	0.8 [0.5, 1.4]	0.9 [0.6, 1.5]

[a] adjusted for maternal age and deprivation.

Association of social and lifestyle factors with fetal and neonatal death from 20 weeks gestation in babies of women with type 1 and type 2 diabetes				
Social and lifestyle factor	Cases n/N (%)	Controls n/N (%)	Crude OR [95% CI]	Adjusted OR[a]
Unplanned pregnancy	40/88 (45)	55/144 (38)	1.4 [0.8, 2.3]	1.3 [0.7, 2.4]
No contraceptive use in the 12 months before pregnancy	49/72 (68)	54/121 (45)	2.6 [1.4, 5.0]	2.5 [1.3, 4.8]
No folic acid commenced prior to pregnancy	48/74 (65)	66/131 (50)	1.8 [1.0, 3.3]	2.0 [1.1, 3.7]
Smoking	43/115 (37)	44/182 (24)	1.9 [0.1, 3.1]	2.1 [1.2, 3.6]
Assessment of suboptimal approach of the woman to managing her diabetes before pregnancy	83/98 (85)	88/154 (57)	4.2 [2.1, 8.1]	4.7 [2.3, 9.3]
Assessment of suboptimal approach of the woman to managing her diabetes during pregnancy	76/124 (61)	56/207 (27)	4.3 [2.6, 7.1]	3.9 [2.4, 6.5]

[a] adjusted for maternal age and deprivation.

Association of glycaemic control factors with fetal and neonatal death from 20 weeks gestation in babies of women with type 1 and type 2 diabetes				
Glycaemic control factor	Cases n/N (%)	Controls n/N (%)	Crude OR [95% CI]	Adjusted OR[a]
No test of glycaemic control before pregnancy	25/90 (28)	24/139 (17)	1.8 [1.0, 3.5]	1.8 [0.9, 3.4]
No local targets set for glycaemic control	31/61 (51)	28/86 (33)	2.1 [1.1, 4.3]	2.1 [1.0, 4.4]
Assessment of suboptimal preconception glycaemic control	103/115 (90)	115/167 (69)	3.9 [1.9, 7.9]	4.3 [2.1, 8.7]
Assessment of suboptimal 1st trimester glycaemic control	109/129 (85)	118/192 (61)	3.4 [1.9, 6.1]	3.4 [1.9, 6.1]
Assessment of suboptimal glycaemic control after 1st trimester	96/133 (72)	76/209 (37)	4.5 [2.7, 7.5]	5.0 [3.0, 8.4]
Assessment of suboptimal blood glucose control during labour and delivery	47/101 (47)	94/202 (47)	1.0 [0.6, 1.6]	1.1 [0.7, 1.8]
No intravenous insulin and dextrose during labour and/or delivery	31/133 (26)	31/127 (14)	2.1 [1.2, 3.6]	2.0 [1.2, 3.6]

[a] adjusted for maternal age and deprivation.

Association of preconception care factors in the 12 months prior to pregnancy with fetal and neonatal death from 20 weeks gestation in babies of women with type 1 and type 2 diabetes				
Preconception care factor	Cases n/N (%)	Controls n/N (%)	Crude OR [95% CI]	Adjusted OR[a]
No contraceptive advice provided before pregnancy	18/51 (35)	19/83 (23)	1.8 [0.8, 4.0]	1.8 [0.8, 4.1]
No discussion of the following specific diabetes issues:				
Alcohol	22/49 (45)	19/66 (29)	2.0 [0.9, 4.4]	2.2 [1.0, 5.2]
Diet	13/65 (20)	12/100 (12)	1.8 [0.8, 4.4]	1.9 [0.8, 4.5]
Poor glycaemic control	12/74 (16)	14/117 (12)	1.4 [0.6, 3.3]	1.3 [0.5, 3.0]
Retinopathy	18/50 (36)	25/96 (26)	1.6 [0.8, 3.4]	1.5 [0.7, 3.3]
Nephropathy	20/47 (43)	29/76 (38)	1.2 [0.6, 2.5]	1.0 [0.5, 2.0]
Hypertension	19/46 (41)	23/75 (31)	1.6 [0.7, 3.5]	1.3 [0.6, 3.1]
No discussion of the following pregnancy issues:				
Increased diabetes surveillance	9/81 (11)	7/124 (6)	2.1 [0.7, 5.9]	1.9 [0.6, 5.5]
Increased pregnancy surveillance	9/73 (12)	8/124 (6)	2.0 [0.7, 5.6]	1.8 [0.6, 5.1]
Increased risk of induction	13/51 (25)	14/110 (13)	2.4 [1.0, 5.5]	2.2 [0.9, 5.5]
Possible caesarean section	14/62 (23)	11/110 (10)	2.6 [1.1, 6.3]	2.8 [1.1, 7.3]
Fetal risks in diabetic pregnancy	12/63 (19)	7/114 (6)	3.6 [1.3, 9.9]	3.1 [1.0, 9.6]
No dietetic review	36/84 (43)	42/135 (61)	1.7 [0.9, 2.9]	1.6 [0.9, 3.0]
No assessment of the following diabetes complications in the 12 months prior to pregnancy:				
Baseline retinal examination	23/88 (26)	18/137 (13)	2.3 [1.2, 4.7]	2.4 [1.2, 5.1]
Baseline test of renal function	19/79 (24)	15/133 (11)	2.5 [1.2, 5.3]	2.8 [1.2, 6.2]
Assessment of albuminuria	28/70 (40)	30/109 (28)	1.8 [0.9, 3.3]	1.9 [1.0, 3.8]
Assessment of suboptimal preconception care (excluding glycaemic control	71/84 (85)	80/134 (60)	3.7 [1.8, 7.5]	4.6 [2.2, 9.9]

[a] adjusted for maternal age and deprivation.

Association of diabetes care factors with fetal and neonatal death from 20 weeks gestation in babies of women with type 1 and type 2 diabetes				
Diabetes care factor	Cases n/N (%)	Controls n/N (%)	Crude OR [95% CI]	Adjusted OR[a]
No retinal assessment during 1st trimester or at booking if later	43/120 (36)	49/183 (27)	1.5 [0.9, 2.5]	1.4 [0.8, 2.3]
No referral to ophthalmologist (if retinopathy present)	9/26 (35)	21/44 (48)	0.6 [0.2, 1.6]	0.4 [0.1, 1.3]
No monitoring for nephropathy	27/130 (21)	26/206 (13)	1.8 [1.0, 3.3]	1.8 [1.0, 3.2]
No test of renal function (if nephropathy present)	9/16 (56)	5/14 (36)	2.3 [0.5, 10.7]	2.7 [0.5, 13.8]
Assessment of suboptimal diabetes care during pregnancy	90/128 (70)	112/204 (55)	2.0 [1.2, 3.1]	1.8 [1.1, 3.0]

[a] adjusted for maternal age and deprivation.

Association of maternity care factors with fetal and neonatal death from 20 weeks gestation in babies of women with type 1 and type 2 diabetes				
Maternity care factor	Cases n/N (%)	Controls n/N (%)	Crude OR [95% CI]	Adjusted OR[a]
Assessment of suboptimal fetal monitoring (with antenatal evidence of growth restricted baby)	6/14 (43)	1/11 (9)	7.5 [0.6, 95.5]	4.4 [0.4, 49.9]
Assessment of suboptimal fetal monitoring (with antenatal evidence of fetal size >90th centile)	29/33 (88)	27/73 (37)	15.8 [4.0, 61.5]	18.3 [5.6, 59.6]
No discussion of mode and timing of delivery	11/111 (10)	4/202 (2)	5.45 [1.7, 17.9]	5.0 [1.5, 16.5]
No administration of antenatal corticosteroids[b]	6/14 (43)	12/33 (36)	1.3 [0.4, 4.8]	1.1 [0.3, 4.4]
Assessment of suboptimal maternity care during the antenatal period	91/132 (69)	95/215 (44)	2.8 [1.8, 4.5]	2.9 [1.8, 4.7]
Assessment of suboptimal maternity care during labour and delivery	51/125 (41)	72/213 (34)	1.4 [0.9, 2.1]	1.3 [0.8, 2.2]

[a] Adjusted for maternal age and deprivation.

[b] Analysis restricted to babies delivering from 24+0 to 35+6 weeks gestation and excluding antepartum stillbirths.

Association of postnatal care factors with fetal and neonatal death from 20 weeks gestation in babies of women with type 1 and type 2 diabetes				
Postnatal care factor	Cases n/N (%)	Controls n/N (%)	Crude OR [95% CI]	Adjusted OR[a]
No postnatal contraceptive advice	41/89 (46)	26/163 (16)	4.5 [2.4, 8.4]	4.8 [2.6, 9.0]
No written plan for post-delivery diabetes management	20/120 (17)	25/188 (13)	1.3 [0.7, 2.5]	1.4 [0.7, 2.8]
Assessment of suboptimal postnatal diabetes care	86/127 (68)	106/211 (50)	2.1 [1.3, 3.3]	2.1 [1.3, 3.5]

[a] adjusted for maternal age and deprivation.

Appendix E

Association between demographic and clinical characteristics, social and lifestyle issues, and clinical care with fetal and neonatal deaths (excluding major fetal congenital anomaly) from 20 weeks of gestation up to 28 days after delivery in babies of women with type 1 and type 2 diabetes

Association between demographic characteristics of fetal and neonatal deaths (excluding major fetal congenital anomaly) from 20 weeks gestation in babies of women with type 1 and type 2 diabetes

Demographic characteristic	Cases n/N (%)	Controls n/N (%)	Crude OR [95% CI]	Adjusted OR
Age	-	-	1.0 [1.0, 1.0]	1.0 [1.0, 1.0][b]
Black, Asian or Other Ethnic Minority group	25/95 (26)	41/220 (19)	1.6 [0.9, 2.8]	1.3 [0.7, 2.5][a]
Primigravidity	48/95 (51)	92/220 (42)	1.4 [0.9, 2.3]	1.5 [0.9, 2.7][a]
Maternal social deprivation[d]	-	-	1.2 [1.0, 1.4]	1.2 [1.0, 1.5][c]

[a] adjusted for maternal age and deprivation.

[b] adjusted for maternal deprivation.

[c] adjusted for maternal age. Odds ratio is for one year increase in maternal age.

[d] Quintile of social deprivation derived from postcode of residence. Odds ratio is for unit increase in deprivation quintile.

Association between clinical characteristics of fetal and neonatal deaths (excluding major fetal congenital anomaly) from 20 weeks gestation in babies of women with type 1 and type 2 diabetes

Clinical characteristic	Cases n/N (%)	Controls n/N (%)	Crude OR [95% CI]	Adjusted OR[a]
Body Mass Index (BMI ≥ 30)	13/56 (23)	33/137 (24)	1.0 [0.5, 2.0]	0.8 [0.3, 1.7]
Pre-existing diabetes complications	15/78 (19)	16/197 (8)	2.7 [1.3, 5.8]	2.1 [0.9, 4.8]
Retinopathy in pregnancy	21/61 (34)	50/167 (30)	1.2 [0.7, 2.3]	1.3 [0.7, 2.6]
Diabetic nephropathy in pregnancy	14/71 (20)	14/185 (8)	3.0 [1.3, 6.8]	2.6 [1.1, 6.1]
Recurrent episodes of hypoglycaemia during pregnancy	42/86 (49)	105/205 (51)	0.9 [0.6, 1.5]	1.1 [0.6, 1.9]
Severe hypoglycaemia during pregnancy (one or more episodes of hypoglycaemia requiring external help)	13/66 (20)	32/167 (19)	1.0 [0.5, 2.1]	1.2 [0.5, 2.6]
Antenatal evidence of fetal growth restriction	11/81 (14)	11/218 (5)	3.0 [1.2, 7.2]	3.0 [1.2, 7.5]
Antenatal evidence of macrosomia (fetal size >90th centile)	32/79 (41)	76/216 (35)	1.3 [0.7, 2.1]	1.4 [0.8, 2.4]

[a] Adjusted for maternal age and deprivation.

Association between social and lifestyle factors of fetal and neonatal deaths (excluding major fetal congenital anomaly) from 20 weeks gestation in babies of women with type 1 and type 2 diabetes

Social and lifestyle factor	Cases n/N (%)	Controls n/N (%)	Crude OR [95% CI]	Adjusted OR[a]
Unplanned pregnancy	29/66 (44)	55/144 (38)	1.3 [0.7, 2.3]	1.2 [0.6, 2.3]
No contraceptive use in the 12 months before pregnancy	38/53 (72)	54/121 (45)	3.1 [1.5, 6.5]	2.7 [1.3, 5.8]
No folic acid commenced prior to pregnancy	34/51 (67)	66/131 (50)	2.0 [1.0, 3.9]	2.1 [1.0, 4.4]
Smoking	28/80 (35)	44/182 (24)	1.7 [1.0, 3.0]	1.7 [0.9, 3.2]
Assessment of suboptimal approach of the woman to managing her diabetes before pregnancy	57/67 (85)	88/154 (57)	4.3 [2.0, 9.3]	4.8 [2.1, 10.7]
Assessment of suboptimal approach of the woman to managing her diabetes during pregnancy	56/87 (64)	56/207 (27)	4.9 [2.8, 8.6]	4.4 [2.5, 7.8]

[a] Adjusted for maternal age and deprivation

Association between glycaemic control factors of fetal and neonatal deaths (excluding major fetal congenital anomaly) from 20 weeks gestation in babies of women with type 1 and type 2 diabetes

Glycaemic control factor	Cases n/N (%)	Controls n/N (%)	Crude OR [95% CI]	Adjusted OR[a]
No test of glycaemic control before pregnancy	18/63 (29)	24/139 (17)	1.9 [0.9, 3.9]	1.9 [0.9, 4.0]
No evidence of local targets set for glycaemic control	24/47 (51)	28/86 (33)	2.2 [1.0, 4.6]	2.2 [1.0, 4.9]
Assessment of suboptimal preconception glycaemic control	69/76 (91)	115/167 (69)	4.5 [1.9, 10.6]	4.8 [2.0, 11.6]
Assessment of suboptimal 1st trimester glycaemic control	77/89 (87)	118/192 (61)	4.0 [2.0, 8.1]	3.9 [1.9, 7.8]
Assessment of suboptimal glycaemic control after 1st trimester	68/93 (73)	76/209 (37)	4.8 [2.7, 8.4]	5.1 [2.9, 9.1]
Assessment of suboptimal blood glucose control during labour and delivery	35/70 (50)	94/202 (47)	1.2 [0.7, 2.0]	1.2 [0.7, 2.2]
No intravenous insulin and dextrose during labour and/or delivery	21/93 (23)	31/127 (14)	1.8 [0.9, 3.3]	1.8 [0.9, 3.4]

[a] Adjusted for maternal age and deprivation.

Association between preconception care factors in the 12 months prior to pregnancy of fetal and neonatal deaths (excluding major fetal congenital anomaly) from 20 weeks gestation in babies of women with type 1 and type 2 diabetes

Preconception care factor	Cases n/N (%)	Controls n/N (%)	Crude OR [95% CI]	Adjusted OR[a]
No contraceptive advice provided before pregnancy	12/36 (33)	19/83 (23)	1.7 [0.7, 4.0]	1.6 [0.7, 3.8]
No discussion of the following specific diabetes issues:				
Alcohol	16/34 (47)	19/66 (29)	2.2 [0.9, 5.3]	2.7 [1.1, 6.9]
Diet	10/47 (21)	12/100 (12)	2.0 [0.8, 5.0]	2.1 [0.8, 5.4]
Poor glycaemic control	10/52 (19)	14/117 (12)	1.8 [0.7, 4.3]	1.6 [0.7, 4.0]
Retinopathy	14/33 (42)	25/96 (26)	2.1 [0.9, 4.9]	2.0 [0.8, 4.7]
Nephropathy	15/34 (44)	29/76 (38)	1.3 [0.6, 2.9]	1.2 [0.5, 2.8]
Hypertension	15/32 (47)	23/75 (31)	2.0 [0.8, 4.7]	1.7 [0.7, 4.3]
No discussion of the following pregnancy issues:				
Increased diabetes surveillance	8/62 (13)	7/124 (6)	2.5 [0.8, 7.3]	2.3 [0.8, 6.8]
Increased pregnancy surveillance	8/55 (15)	8/124 (6)	2.5 [0.9, 7.0]	2.2 [0.8, 6.5]
Increased risk of induction	11/40 (28)	14/110 (13)	2.6 [1.1, 6.5]	2.3 [0.9, 6.2]
Possible caesarean section	13/46 (28)	11/110 (10)	3.6 [1.4, 8.9]	3.7 [1.4, 10.2]
Fetal risks in diabetic pregnancy	10/46 (22)	7/114 (6)	4.3 [1.5, 12.4]	3.6 [1.1, 11.6]
No dietetic review	22/60 (37)	42/135 (61)	1.3 [0.7, 2.4]	1.3 [0.6, 2.5]
No assessment of the following diabetes complications in the 12 months prior to pregnancy:				
Baseline retinal examination	17/61 (28)	18/137 (13)	2.6 [1.2, 5.5]	2.6 [1.2, 5.9]
Baseline test of renal function	14/58 (24)	15/133 (11)	2.5 [1.1, 5.7]	2.6 [1.1, 6.3]
Assessment of albuminuria	19/54 (35)	30/109 (28)	1.4 [0.7, 2.9]	1.6 [0.8, 3.3]
Assessment of suboptimal preconception care (excluding glycaemic control)	48/58 (83)	80/134 (60)	3.2 [1.5, 7.1]	4.0 [0.7, 9.4]

[a] Adjusted for maternal age and deprivation.

Association between diabetes care factors of fetal and neonatal deaths (excluding major fetal congenital anomaly) from 20 weeks gestation in babies of women with type 1 and type 2 diabetes

Diabetes care factor	Cases n/N (%)	Controls n/N (%)	Crude OR [95% CI]	Adjusted OR[a]
	27/83 (33)	49/183 (27)	1.3 [0.8, 2.3]	1.2 [0.7, 2.2]
No referral to ophthalmologist (if retinopathy present)	6/16 (38)	21/44 (48)	0.7 [0.2, 2.2]	0.6 [0.2, 2.3]
No monitoring for nephropathy	19/91 (21)	26/206 (13)	1.8 [1.0, 3.5]	1.8 [0.9, 3.5]
No test of renal function (if nephropathy present)	8/14 (58)	5/14 (36)	2.4 [0.5, 11.7]	2.9 [0.5, 15.8]
Assessment of suboptimal diabetes care during pregnancy	67/91 (74)	112/204 (55)	2.3 [1.3, 4.0]	2.2 [1.3, 3.9]

[a] Adjusted for maternal age and deprivation.

Association between maternity care factors of fetal and neonatal deaths (excluding major fetal congenital anomaly) from 20 weeks gestation in babies of women with type 1 and type 2 diabetes

Maternity care factor	Cases n/N (%)	Controls n/N (%)	Crude OR [95% CI]	Adjusted OR[a]
Assessment of suboptimal fetal monitoring (with antenatal evidence of growth restricted baby)	5/11 (45)	1/11 (9)	8.3 [0.6, 119.3]	5.2 [0.4, 62.8]
Assessment of suboptimal fetal monitoring (with antenatal evidence of fetal size >90th centile)	28/32 (88)	27/73 (37)	15.2 [3.9, 59.2]	17.7 [5.4, 57.6]
No discussion of mode and timing of delivery	9/79 (12)	4/202 (2)	6.7 [1.9, 23.0]	5.9 [1.7, 20.7]
No administration of antenatal corticosteroids[b]	2/7 (29)	12/33 (36)	0.7 [0.1, 4.3]	0.4 [0.0, 4.1]
Assessment of suboptimal maternity care during the antenatal period	68/90 (76)	95/215 (44)	3.9 [2.2, 7.0]	4.2 [2.3, 7.4]
Assessment of suboptimal maternity care during labour and delivery	34/88 (39)	72/213 (34)	1.2 [0.7, 2.1]	1.2 [0.7, 2.1]

[a] Adjusted for maternal age and deprivation.

[b] Analysis restricted to babies delivering from 24+0 to 35+6 weeks gestation and excluding antepartum stillbirths.

Association between postnatal care factors of fetal and neonatal deaths (excluding major fetal congenital anomaly) from 20 weeks gestation in babies of women with type 1 and type 2 diabetes

Postnatal care factor	Cases n/N (%)	Controls n/N (%)	Crude OR [95% CI]	Adjusted OR[a]
No postnatal contraceptive advice	24/60 (40)	26/163 (16)	3.5 [1.8, 7.0]	4.1 [2.0, 8.2]
No written plan for post-delivery diabetes management	12/84 (14)	25/188 (13)	1.1 [0.5, 2.3]	1.2 [0.5, 2.6]
Assessment of suboptimal postnatal diabetes care	61/87 (70)	106/211 (50)	2.3 [1.4, 4.0]	2.5 [1.4, 4.3]

[a] Adjusted for maternal age and deprivation.

Appendix F - CEMACH advisory groups & contributors

Appendix F - CEMACH advisory groups & contributors

Diabetes Professional Advisory Group

Stephen Walkinshaw	Chair, Consultant Obstetrician, Liverpool Women's Hospital
Jean Chapple	Consultant in Perinatal Epidemiology, Westminster Primary Care Trust
Richard Congdon	CEMACH Chief Executive
Simon Court	Consultant Paediatrician, Newcastle General Hospital (Diabetes UK)
Pat Doyle	Epidemiologist, London School of Hygiene & Tropical Medicine
Kate Fleming	CEMACH Senior Data Analyst (until November 2006)
Shona Golightly	CEMACH Director of Development and Research
Olwen Harrison	Diabetes Nurse Specialist, North Hampshire Hospital
Jane Hawdon	Consultant Neonatologist, University College London Hospitals
Gillian Hawthorne	Consultant Diabetes Physician, Newcastle General Hospital
Anita Holdcroft	Consultant Anaesthetist, Chelsea and Westminster Hospital, London
Julie Maddocks	CEMACH Regional Manager (North West & West Midlands)
Mary Macintosh	CEMACH Medical Director (Until May 2006)
Rona McCandlish	Professor of Midwifery, National Perinatal Epidemiology Unit
Jo Modder	CEMACH Clinical Director (Obstetrics)
Alison Miller	CEMACH Programme Director and Midwifery Lead
Mary Pierce	Royal College of General Practitioners representative
Bob Young	Consultant Diabetes Physician, Hope Hospital, Salford

CEMACH Central Office Staff

Dominique Acolet	Clinical Director (Perinatal Epidemiology)
Naufil Alam	Data Analyst
Jessica Berenston-Shaw	National Clinical Projects Advisor
John Bolton	Accountant
Nicola Cogdell	Administrative Assistant
Kirshnee Chetty	Administrative Assistant (until February 2007)
Richard Congdon	Chief Executive
Shona Golightly	Director of Research and Development
Rosie Houston	Assistant Projects Manager
Mary Humphreys	Office Administrator
Alison Miller	Programme Director and Midwifery Lead
Jo Modder	Clinical Director (Obstetrics)
Iman Mortagy	Data Analyst
Dharmishta Parmar	Data Manager
Gale Pearson	Clinical Director (Child Health)
Maureen Wilson	Committee Administrator

CEMACH Regional Managers

Lesley Anson	Yorkshire & Humberside (until March 2006)
Angela Bell	Northern Ireland
Melanie Gompels	South East and the Channel Islands
Carol Hay	East of England
Julie Maddocks	North West / West Midlands
Marjorie Renwick	North East
Dawn Roberts	Wales
Rachel Thomas	London
Rosie Thompson	South West
Sue Wood	East Midlands and Yorkshire & Humberside

Panel Chairs

Carol Axon	Midwife, South West
Philip Banfield	Consultant Obstetrician, Wales
Miriam Bonduelle	Consultant Obstetrician, Wales
Ian Casson	Consultant Physician, North West
Jean Chapple	Consultant in Perinatal Epidemiology, London
Elizabeth Draper	Senior Research Fellow in Reproductive and Paediatric Epidemiology, East Midlands
D A Evans	Consultant Obstetrician, North East
Robert Fraser	Reader in Reproductive & Developmental Medicine, Consultant in Obstetrics & Gynaecology, Yorkshire & Humberside
Malcolm Griffiths	Consultant Obstetrician & Gynaecologist, East of England
Paul Jennings	Consultant Physician in Diabetes and Endocrinology, Yorkshire & Humberside
Boon Lim	Consultant Obstetrician, East of England
Michael Maresh	Consultant Obstetrician, North West
Heulwen Morgan	Consultant Obstetrician, London
C M Ritchie	Consultant Physician, Northern Ireland
A I Traub	Consultant Obstetrician, Northern Ireland
Matthew Coleman	Consultant Obstetrician, South East
Michael Gillmer	Consultant Obstetrician, South East
Andrew Johnson	Consultant Physician, South West
Michael Quinn	Consultant Paediatrician, South West
Dorothea Smith	Midwife, South East
Derek Tuffnell	Consultant Obstetrician, Yorkshire & Humberside
Christopher Watts	Director of Public Health, London
Sarah Wilson	Director of Public Health, East Midlands
Christopher Wright	Consultant Perinatal Pathologist, North East

CEMACH Board

Michael Weindling	Chair
Jean Chapple	Faculty of Public Health
Griselda Cooper	Royal College of Anaesthetists
Beverley Fitzsimons	Lay representative
Steve Gould	Royal College of Pathologists
Ian Greer	Chair, CEMACH National Advisory Committee for Maternal Health
Sheila Hollins	Royal College of Psychiatrists
Deirdre Kelly	Chair, CEMACH National Advisory Committee for Child Health
Jenni McAughey	Chair of RCGP Northern Ireland Council
Neil McIntosh	Royal College of Paediatrics and Child Health
Ann Seymour	Lay representative
Louise Silverton	Royal College of Midwives
Allan Templeton	Royal College of Obstetricians & Gynaecologists
Una Rennard	Lay representative

Diabetes Enquiry Panel Assessors (can be accessed at www.cemach.org.uk)

Diabetes Multidisciplinary Resource Group (can be accessed at www.cemach.org.uk)